The GASTROPARESIS Healing Diet

A Guided Program for Promoting Gastric Relief, Reducing Symptoms and Feeling Great

Tammy Chang

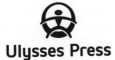

Ulysses Press

Dedicated to the gastroparesis community

Published in the United States by:
Ulysses Press
P.O. Box 3440
Berkeley, CA 94703
www.ulyssespress.com

ISBN13: 978-1-61243-645-6
Library of Congress Control Number: 2016950672

Printed in the United States by United Graphics Inc.
10 9 8 7 6 5 4 3 2 1

Acquisitions Editor: Casie Vogel
Managing Editor: Claire Chun
Editor: Renee Rutledge
Proofreader: Shayna Keyles
Index: Sayre Van Young
Front cover/interior design: what!design @ whatweb.com
Layout: Jake Flaherty
Cover artwork: © Lesterman/shutterstock.com

Distributed by Publishers Group West

CONTENTS

INTRODUCTION

Welcome! My name is Tammy, and I am a nutrition coach and cook based in the San Francisco Bay Area. Chances are you are here because you've been diagnosed with something called gastroparesis (GP), and you are unsure where to start. You may be feeling a bit overwhelmed at the moment. Perhaps you've done a bit of research online, and it's possible you aren't feeling so excited about the path that lies ahead of you.

I'm glad you are here. As I've delved into the world of gastroparesis, I have spoken with many courageous individuals, from those who have had many medical interventions to those who merely need to remove some problematic foods from their diets. There is a very large spectrum of experience with GP, and depending on where you may fall, you have a small to large job ahead of you.

One comforting aspect is that you aren't alone. Since GP is just beginning to be more widely recognized as a disease, there aren't many accurate statistics. At the very least, there are tens of thousands of diagnosed cases, and as it starts to become a more recognized digestive disorder, numbers will only become more accurate. At the time of this writing, one of the well-known Facebook support groups has almost 10,000 members, many of which are active, supportive members of the GP community.

I personally do not have gastroparesis, so when my publisher asked me if I was interested in creating recipes for the GP community, I was a little hesitant. At the time, I knew very little besides what I had often heard for those with slow motility: eat low-fat low-fiber foods (fat and fiber are two things that tend to take longer to digest). My publisher was convinced that my nutrition advice would be helpful, so I decided to take on the project.

As I started to research gastroparesis, I found myself feeling overwhelmed. One statistic I read said that 1 in 10 patients diagnosed have severe enough symptoms to greatly impact quality of life.[1] This disease can be debilitating, and for some of you, it will be a reason why your life cannot be the same as it was before. However, I found that the GP community, along with its taking in people's harder days, is also extremely loving, supportive, and strong.

As I witnessed many people reaching out for help online, I had much self-doubt. How can I offer those with gastroparesis something valuable, without myself having this condition?

Then I began interviewing and talking with those with GP (I'll refer to them as GPers from here) and was blessed to be connected with wonderful people, many of whom were dealing with their symptoms on a daily basis and still finding the energy to advocate and educate others about GP. Each person had some beautiful insight that helped shape my outlook and mold the contents of this book, which would not have been possible without their input and inspiration. Some have chosen to remain anonymous, and some are leaders in the GP community with their own blogs and advocacy work, whom I hope you will continue to learn from and support as they fight for understanding and for your rights. Their stories and words of wisdom are scattered throughout the book in the "Personal Insight" sections.

As I listened and learned, I realized that I have some things to share with you, and the content for this book began to take shape. When

1 "Gastroparesis," National Organization for Rare Disorders, last modified 2012, accessed August 5, 2016, http://rarediseases.org/rare-diseases/gastroparesis.

working with clients, I always look at starting from one place and reaching somewhere different. Armed with the right information about how to nourish body and soul, anyone can start with small steps and move forward to the best of their capabilities. This book will examine how you can do those things. Right now, you might not have an idea of what is possible: how active you can be, what foods you can eat, or how much you can eat at one time. I'll cover how to tackle all of that.

I'll also talk about what gastroparesis does, and look at some of the reasons why it is such a complicated matter, so that you can understand why it's a completely individual experience for anyone who is diagnosed with GP.

This book is also a chance for me to share what I know about holistic nutrition and making simple food taste really darn good. There are some very simple recipes in this book that are based on nutrient-dense, whole foods. You first have to figure out what works for you, and then you'll have a strong foundation from which to add.

The Gastroparesis Healing Diet is also a guide to understanding what your body needs when it comes to nutrition. Here, I'll offer some tips and ideas on how to begin to understand your reactions and create an awareness around your health that may not have been there before. A diagnosis of gastroparesis should make this goal your first priority.

Hopefully this journey will bring some new resources to you and expand your community in new and powerful ways, just as writing this book has connected me with strong and vibrant individuals who have the desire to strengthen the gastroparesis community and to thrive in the best way they can.

Much of the literature out there says there is no cure for gastroparesis, but there are ways to manage the disease. I've heard a few success stories where people have made huge turnarounds. This may be in your future. However, all of you have a similar journey at this moment, no matter where you are, and it takes a lot of trial and error since everyone's reactions to possible medications and therapies are different. This book is not going to focus on the breadth of different therapies and medications out there. Instead, I will focus on food and what you can do through your lifestyle, day to day.

This book will deal mainly with how to explore a more holistic and nutrition-based approach to gastroparesis-friendly foods. Often, when people have flare-ups, they will rely on products such as Ensure or Pedialyte, which at times can be necessary, but also come with a lot of artificial ingredients. I will talk about the importance of eating clean, and since whole foods–based nutrition exists, then why not nourish yourself in that way?

Figuring out how to live vibrantly with GP requires a multifaceted approach to reducing any possible stressors and making sure that all parts of self-care are at their ideal level. This way, the body can heal and function at its best.

GETTING STARTED

How should you read this book? Well, there is a lot of information here, some of which is pretty scientific and will help you understand more about what is happening inside your body. This is important, because you *will* have to self-advocate, and knowing what is going on inside your body and correlating that with what you may be experiencing is helpful.

However, if you are feeling overwhelmed at the moment and you want to get to creating a plan, then jump to Chapter 3.

It will be helpful to look at your state of mind before you start. It's very possible that you may not have the energy to be the person you were in a previous time of your life. Perhaps you are attached to this former version of yourself. In many interviews, the idea of needing to relearn your body comes up: to relearn what you can eat, to relearn how much energy you can expend, and to relearn how much responsibility to take on. During the interview process, I had to reschedule multiple times with people, because sometimes they just didn't feel well enough to speak, or they had to have an emergency procedure. This can be a tough transition time, because you may be putting expectations upon yourself that an able-bodied person would have. More than one mother expressed that they had to deal with the guilt of not being the mom they wanted to be. We all have to learn to be gentle with ourselves, and you more than most.

One helpful way to think about daily living with chronic illness is called the Spoon Theory. The Spoon Theory was created by Christine Miserandino when one of her best friends asked her what it was like to live with lupus. Many people with chronic illness find the Spoon Theory relatable and helpful for explaining to healthy, able-bodied friends what daily living is like with a chronic illness. Essentially, each spoon is a unit of energy that you have. A healthy person seems to have an unlimited number of spoons; they rarely have to make choices about what they can do energy-wise during the day. However, for someone living with chronic illness, it's perhaps either washing the dishes or doing the laundry, but not both.

As you come to understand your body and the way it responds to gastroparesis and the demands of your daily life, you'll start to understand how many spoons you have day to day, how things fluctuate, and how much you need to slow down and take care of yourself.

Chapter 1
WHAT IS GASTROPARESIS?

You don't realize how much your stomach does for you until it stops doing what it's supposed to. Ideally, food moves through the stomach to the small intestine on its own, through a process called gastric emptying by involuntary (meaning you don't think about it) muscle contractions.

If we break down the word, "gastro" means of or relating to the stomach, and "paresis" means a condition of muscular weakness caused by nerve damage or disease. "Gastroparesis" literally means muscular weakness of the stomach that is caused by nerve damage or disease. When you first start to research GP, the most commonly cited reason you'll find for the disease is that there is damage to the vagus nerve. The vagus nerve is a cranial nerve that extends from the brain and through the abdomen through many different organs. It is responsible for many actions in the body, motility being one of them. However, the vagus nerve is only one possible culprit for causing gastroparesis. Thus, the above definition only partially does gastroparesis justice, mainly because there are most likely other causes that can decrease the motility in the stomach.

Gastroparesis is essentially a motility disease. Motility refers to the movement of food through your digestive system. Motility is aided by smooth muscle contractions throughout the digestive system. Throughout the book I will use the term interchangeably with peristalsis, which refers to the smooth muscle contractions specifically.

Gastroparesis is just one of the many digestive diseases that afflict at least 60 to 70 million people in the US; that's the number of reported cases of digestive diseases from a 2009 NIH report.[2] You could also think of that as all the people living in France. Gastroparesis, however, is considered a rare disease, since fewer than 200,000 people in the US are diagnosed with it.

Exact numbers for gastroparesis are not entirely accurate, since this is still a disease becoming more well-known. One source reports that there are 24.2 reported cases among 100,000 people, which, if you figure that the US population is around 320 million, is 76,800 people.[3] This is a small number, for instance, compared to the 2.8 million women who either currently have breast cancer or have some history with the disease, according to Breastcancer.org.[4] With higher numbers, more awareness and research follow. Many GPers struggle with the fact that few people have heard of GP, including their own doctors. The good news is there are those who are advocating for more awareness and support, some of whom you'll be introduced to later!

Currently, gastroparesis is diagnosed by a test that measures the time it takes for the stomach to empty, called gastric emptying scintigraphy. You most likely have taken this exact test. Usually an egg or egg substitute is served with a bit of radioactive material and then tracked to see how long it takes for the stomach to empty. If more

2 National Institute of Diabetes and Digestive and Kidney Diseases, "Digestive Diseases Statistics for the United States," National Institutes of Health, September 2013, Accessed July 23, 2016, https://www.niddk.nih.gov/health-information/health-statistics/Documents/Digestive_Disease_Stats_508.pdf.

3 Enrique Ray, et al., "Prevalence of Hidden Gastroparesis in the Community," *Journal of Neurogastroenterol Motility* 18, no. 1 (January 18, 2012). DOI: 10.5056/jnm.2012.18.1.34.

4 "US Breast Cancer Statistics," BreastCancer.org, last modified September 30, 2016, accessed October 1, 2016, http://www.breastcancer.org/symptoms/understand_bc/statistics.

than 10 percent of the meal is still in the stomach after four hours, a diagnosis of gastroparesis is given.[5]

Since gastroparesis is still largely unknown, there isn't a standard diagnosis for the different types. If the delay is mild, it can also be called functional dyspepsia or non-ulcer dyspepsia.

Although not completely put into practice, there is a proposed grading system for severity.

Grade 1: Mild GP	Symptoms relatively easy to control. Able to maintain weight and nutrition on a modified diet.
Grade 2: Compensated GP	Moderate symptoms with partial control through use of pharmacological agents. Able to maintain nutrition with dietary and lifestyle adjustments. Rare hospital admissions.
Grade 3: Severe GP	Persistent symptoms despite medical intervention. Inability to maintain nutrition through oral intake of food. Frequent emergency room visits or hospitalizations.

As you can see from the adapted chart[6] above, this can be extremely uncomfortable and upsetting at any grade. To what degree depends on the person. It's also possible to have very slow gastric emptying but not exhibit that many symptoms. Common symptoms of GP are:

- Nausea

- Rapid fullness at the beginning of meals

- Abdominal bloating

- Abdominal pain

---

5 Pataramon Vasavid, et al., "Normal Solid Gastric Emptying Values Measured by Scintigraphy Using Asian-Style Meal: A Multicenter Study in Healthy Volunteers," *Journal of Neurogastroenterology and Motility* 20, no. 3 (June 20, 2014), DOI: 10.5056/JMN13115.

6 Shamaila Waseem, et al., "Gastroparesis: Current Diagnostic Challenges and Management Considerations," *World Journal of Gastroenterology* 15, no. 1 (January 7, 2009). DOI: 10.3748/WJG.15.25.

- Acid reflux

- Weight loss

- Loss of appetite

- Blood sugar swings

- Fatigue

- Belching

- Malnutrition

It's also not uncommon for those with gastroparesis to be diagnosed with other gastrointestinal ailments and chronic illness. For those more severely afflicted, a combination of things can be happening that affect the body.

One condition I kept reading about is the possibility of bezoars, which is essentially a collection of undigested food, with either high cellulose content or other indigestible fibers, that can create blockages in the GI tract. According to Rarediseases.org, bezoars are a rare occurrence for those with gastroparesis, although because of delayed stomach emptying, you might be at higher risk. When they do occur, they don't always cause problems, but are taken care of either through dissolving with chemicals, removing endoscopically, or in more severe cases, surgery.

Many women also find that their menstrual cycles greatly affect their symptoms. We'll talk more about the exact mechanisms behind this in Chapter 3. I've learned from my interviews that I can't stress enough that everyone experiences gastroparesis differently; some find it mildly discomforting, and others find that it dramatically impacts their quality of life and ability to work. One common thread, however, is that with trial and error, people find what little tricks and ways of eating work for them.

WHAT CAUSES GASTROPARESIS?

One of the best sites I've seen summarizing gastroparesis causes and treatments is Rarediseases.org. They emphasize that gastroparesis "is a complex, multifactor, chronic, digestive disease state with possible genetic, physiological, immune, psychological, social, and environmental interplays."[7]

We are working with many unknowns when it comes to gastroparesis, and there are always different factors that come into play when the disease finally manifests itself.

One of the known major causes of gastroparesis is diabetes, where high blood sugar can cause damage to the nerves that control stomach muscle contraction. Other causes can be viral infections or other diseases that damage nerves and muscles, like scleroderma and Parkinson's. In some cases, a cause is currently unknown and labeled idiopathic.

The same site tells of a clinic that surveyed its 146 GP patients. Of those 146 patients, they found that 36 percent were idiopathic, 29 percent were diabetic, 13 percent were post-surgical, 7.5 percent had Parkinson's disease, and 4.8 percent had collagen diseases.[8]

Let's take a moment to discuss idiopathic cases. One of the interviewees, Sam (you'll find his wisdom on page 58), shares the idea that often, idiopathic cases do have a cause. Western medicine is great at treating symptoms and prolonging life, but it doesn't always look around to find the root cause. The fact that it labels certain cases idiopathic doesn't mean that GP came up out of nowhere. It's important to look at your health holistically, and if your case is idiopathic, then question what might be causing your gastroparesis and make changes accordingly.

---

7 "Gastroparesis," National Organization for Rare Disorders, last modified 2012, accessed August 5, 2016, http://rarediseases.org/rare-diseases/gastroparesis.
8 Ibid.

When I go through the anatomy of the stomach in the next chapter, you'll begin to see that there are many areas in the stomach that can be compromised, and that there are numerous factors that could be affecting it.

WHO IS DIAGNOSED WITH GASTROPARESIS?

Gastroparesis is biased toward women, with 80 percent of idiopathic cases occurring in females. The average age of onset is 34 years,[9] but it can affect anyone at any age. Both type 1 and type 2 diabetes patients make up a large percentage of those diagnosed. Also, post-surgical patients who have had some work done in the trunk and abdomen can experience damage to the vagus nerve and experience delayed gastric emptying.

TREATMENT OPTIONS

It is not within the scope of this book to discuss all the treatment options available and in trial for GP. I'll discuss some of the basic ones. Depending on the severity of your GP, the dietary suggestions in this book will be more effective after you have worked with a knowledgeable medical professional to figure out what medications or interventions are best suited for you.

The most basic medications help to speed up motility and are called *prokinetics*. They primarily work by blocking dopamine receptors, which slow down gastric emptying and motility.[10] The two most common medications are metoclopramide (Reglan) and domperidone (Motilium). Domperidone is not currently FDA approved, but there

9 "What is Gastroparesis?" gastroparesisclinic.org, accessed July 10, 2016, http://www.gastroparesisclinic.org/index.php?pageId=1149&moduleId=195.

10 JE Valenzuela, et al., "Dopamine Antagonists in the Upper Gastrointestinal Tract," *Scandinavian Journal of Gastroenterology*, Supplement (1984), Accessed September 15, 2016, http://www.ncbi.nlm.nih.gov/pubmed/6382574.

is acknowledgment by the FDA that some gastrointestinal illnesses might benefit from domperidone, even though there can be serious side effects, especially for those who have cardiac problems. Your doctor can petition for its use on the FDA website.

Reglan has severe side effects, one of which is tardive dyskinesia, an involuntary muscle movement that has the potential to become permanent. More than one interviewee has had this happen to them. As with any medication, it should be taken with care.

Other medications that can be taken in conjunction with prokinetics are *antiemetics*, which help to alleviate nausea, a very common symptom.

With any medication, there is always a risk of side effects. Depending on what else is happening for you, some medications may simply be a bad idea. This is where having a knowledgeable physician and gastroenterologist is extremely important. Fully understanding the pros and cons of each medication, plus having the mindset that they may or may not work for you, is important when trying to find an effective treatment protocol.

As GP gets more severe, some surgical interventions can greatly improve symptoms and help with malnutrition. It's equally important to find good surgeons and doctors that are familiar with these procedures and their risks and potential benefits.

I've included some resources on page 167 that provide better insight into the treatment options available for you, if you should need them.

Personal Insight
Trish, 38, North Carolina

Trish has had many surgical medical interventions that have helped her survive and continue with her advocacy work with GP. Trish's tips for finding the best medical care are invaluable.

Tell us your diagnosis story.

I had been sick nonstop starting in February 2013. I was unable to keep anything down at all. I had the norovirus, and to begin with, they thought it was a stomach bug. But it just never got better—it got worse. I had no appetite, and every time I tried to drink or eat, I would vomit or dry heave.

We don't know if the virus was what caused the GP, but it's possible the virus tipped it over. I had symptoms throughout my life, like lack of appetite and nausea. My husband took me to a hospital in Chapel Hill in April, and I was hospitalized for a week and put on liquids. I was diagnosed with GP that April.

What surgical interventions do you have?

I've had a feeding tube since May 2013. Right now I have a G-J tube,[11] and I can vent something if it doesn't agree with me. All of my nutrition comes from my feeding tube. Although, even with the feeding tube, I'm not getting the adequate nutrients.

I had my colon removed in January 2016, and I now have an ileostomy bag.[12]

I also have a PICC line.[13] I get hydration support through an IV three times a week.

Are you still able to eat?

I don't do any solid foods, but I still take in frozen fluids, like sherbet. My stomach doesn't like yogurt, but I try. Even with fluids, I have a lot of pain afterward. I try to take small sips of fluids that work for me throughout the day. Maybe 250 milliliters (1 cup) total, on good days.

---

11 A G-J tube stands for gastro-jejunal tube. One part connects to the stomach, the other connects to the small intestine.

12 An ileostomy is when the small intestine is separated from the large intestine, and the end of the small intestine is connected to the wall of the abdomen to create an opening that connects to an outer bag, called an ileostomy bag. This bag collects wastes from meals and must be emptied several times a day. There are not accurate numbers, but according to the Crohn's and Colitis Foundation of America, it's estimated that 450,000 to 600,000 people are living with an ileostomy bag.

13 A PICC line stands for peripherally inserted central catheter, which is a tube inserted into the arm that can stay there for further use.

What have you found to be helpful in dealing with this disease?

I'm able to keep positive most of the time because I have support from my family. I do see a psychotherapist to try and live with the emotions from chronic illness. It has been helpful. I was reluctant in the beginning because I thought they were trying to tell me that it was all in my head, but it wasn't like that. I was going through a lot of guilt about not being the mom that I wanted to be, and my psychotherapist helped me work through it.

We found that writing and blogging were helpful to get the thoughts out and the load off my back. That's helped a lot. Talking to others online and advocating is helpful as well.

I try to do some stretching and that helps a little bit. That comes and goes. I don't get out of the house as much as I'd like to, but getting out of the house, even if it's to go for a car ride, is helpful.

I try to listen to what my body is saying and not overthink what I'm going through. I don't want to constantly think of what I can't do, and just try and take it moment by moment.

What advice would you give to someone newly diagnosed?

To be patient with your body, because it is a lot of trial and error trying to figure out what works for you and what doesn't. If you are experimenting, limit the things you are trying to do so that you can figure it out. When your body needs to rest, don't be overzealous. Rest. There's a lot of educating yourself about this, but also educating other medical professionals that you run into. Be mindful that you'll have to do this. Find a good support team, whether online or in person. There are times when you'll want someone to understand—even though your family is great, they don't understand that actual experience. Be honest with your doctors about symptoms. They can't help you if they can't understand your experience.

Treatment options right now are very limited. What works for some does not work for others. Having a feeding tube is not the worst thing in your life. I ended up not knowing what I was getting into. It has been a big life change, but it's been a lifesaver as well. Same thing with the ileostomy bag. You can adjust once you see what they can do for you. Be honest with yourself with what you are willing to try and not try.

Thank you so much! Trish's blog is at Gastroparesiscrusader.weebly.com.

Chapter 2
YOUR DIGESTIVE SYSTEM

The digestive system, which breaks down foods into their smallest parts so you can absorb them, is very elaborate and complicated. It's often called the second brain because of the number of nerves that are connected to it. In fact, 70 percent of all of your nerves are interconnected within the digestive system. No wonder it is such a bother when something isn't working right, which is exactly why you are here. No one has to tell you that your day can be ruined by something off in your digestive system.

Later in this chapter, I'll focus specifically on what happens in the stomach alone—and there is a *lot* happening. There are many hormones and different nerve endings that dictate everything that happens in the stomach, such as whether the different parts of the stomach should contract or relax, or what digestive aids should be secreted. Since we are all individual people, any part of this process could be compromised.

I will also discuss things that you can do that have been known to help or hinder digestion and motility. Whether or not these specific things will help you is a matter of trial and error. Let's begin.

Before I can even start talking about the digestive system, it's important to discuss the nervous system.

THE NERVOUS SYSTEM

The nervous system can be defined as a network of nerve cells and fibers that transmit messages to different parts of the body. The difference between parasympathetic and sympathetic mode explains an important connection between the nervous system and digestion.

Many of you have heard of the "fight-or-flight" mode, where people are able to do magnificent and lifesaving feats while trying to save their lives or the lives of others. The fight-or-flight mode is also called the *sympathetic mode*. In the modern day, it is often activated; not because we are running for lives, but because we are so darn busy all the time. In sympathetic mode, there are things your body does to allow you to have as much energy as possible: it raises your blood sugar, increases your heart rate, sends more blood to your limbs, and shuts off functions that do not aid in fight or flight, such as digestion, your immune system, and your reproductive system. This is why gastrointestinal issues are exacerbated by stress.

The *parasympathetic mode* is what can be thought of as the "rest and digest" state. When your nervous system is in this mode, it will enhance your digestion. I would even go as far as saying that it is your parasympathetic system that is mainly responsible for your digestion working properly.

Many of the smooth muscle cells that are responsible for your motility are activated by the parasympathetic mode. Have you ever been really stressed and felt food just sitting in your stomach? That's the reason.

It's also important to note that the immune system and the reproductive system also work in parasympathetic mode.

THE ENTERIC NERVOUS SYSTEM

There are nerves that connect the digestive system to your brain, but most of the body's nerve connections are located among the digestive system organs alone. This is called the enteric nervous system. The ENS is the intrinsic nervous system located within the walls of the digestive system, starting from your esophagus to your anus.

The ENS is significant because it can practically run *independently* from your brain. Due to the ENS, if the nerve endings to your central nervous system were cut, the digestive system would still function.[14] The brain does not tell the digestive system to secrete this and break apart that. It is the ENS that calls the majority of the shots. For this reason, it is often called the "second brain" or the "brain below." In fact, 90% of the nerve fibers in the vagus nerve carry messages from the gut to the brain, not the other way around.[15]

Remember from the introduction that the digestive system has 70 percent of all the body's nerve endings. This is the ENS. It's complicated, and always talking to itself. With gastroparesis, there are a number of places where nerves can be compromised, and possibly hormones as well.

ANATOMY OF THE DIGESTIVE SYSTEM

When you take a bite of an apple, this is the journey it takes.

STEP 1: The mouth. As you chew thoroughly (which is very important), your saliva coats each particle and starts the digestion process. There are enzymes in your saliva that start to work on the carbohydrates in the piece of apple. The smaller you break down pieces of

---

14 "IBS and Serotonin," Canadian Society of Intestinal Research, July/August 2014, Accessed June 23, 2016, http://www.badgut.org/information-centre/a-z-digestive-topics/ibs-and-serotonin.
15 Adam Hadhazy, "Think Twice: How the Gut's 'Second Brain' Influences Mood and Well-being," *Scientific American*, Feb 12, 2010, Accessed Dec. 8, 2016, https://www.scientificamerican.com/article/gut-second-brain.

food in your mouth, the more you will be able to digest and absorb them. You are essentially creating more surface area so that your body can get more nutrients.

STEP 2: The esophagus. This is the last voluntary action that you do. You contract muscles in your neck to swallow the ball of apple, called a *bolus*. The bolus passes through your esophagus, past a flap called the esophageal sphincter that quickly opens and closes, and lands in your stomach. Sometimes this sphincter can be looser than normal and allow food to come back up into the esophagus, leading to heartburn, or gastroesophageal reflux disease (GERD). This is a *very* common problem for gastroparesis sufferers, but other people suffer from it as well; roughly 20 to 30 percent of adults have this every week.

STEP 3: The stomach. I am going to give a bit more attention to the stomach in the second part of this chapter, because this is where delayed emptying occurs. Ideally, this is where the bolus mixes with stomach acid. Proteins and minerals are broken down. The stomach mixes everything together and slowly releases what is now called chyme (food and stomach acid mixed together).

STEP 4: The small intestine. When the chyme passes from the stomach into the small intestine, the pancreas releases special enzymes, which help break down the bits of food even further. The small intestine is lined with little fingers called villi, and they grab on to nutrients and pull them into the bloodstream, where the nutrients are carried to other parts of your body.

STEP 5: The liver. During a meal, your liver also has a job here. It releases something called bile that helps digest your fats. Between meals, bile is stored in your gallbladder and waits until you start eating to do its job. When the chyme enters your small intestine, the bile is released from the gallbladder, and it starts to break down your fats.

STEP 6: The large intestine. Once all the nutrients are absorbed, the leftovers now enter your large intestine, also called your colon. Food moves slower here, and with the help of the billions of bacteria that live in your colon, the food bits are broken down even further to feed your bacteria.

A ton of new research is coming out now about how important these bacteria are. There is a really delicate balance of good and bad bacteria in the body. These bacteria not only help you to further break food down, but they are also responsible for their own secretions, including making some vitamins and helping the immune system. There are things that you can do to support your gut bacteria, which I will talk about in Chapter 4.

Bacteria also produces mucus, which helps move the waste along. If everything is going right, you should be able to rid your body of waste in good time. You don't want waste to hang out too long—that's what we call constipation. One of the functions of your colon is to reabsorb water back into your body, and as your waste hangs out, it becomes more and more compact and harder to pass. Constipation is a common symptom of gastroparesis, and you might have experienced some severe episodes.

THE STOMACH

I've just gone through a very quick, bare-bones view of what happens in your digestive system. The reality, however, is that what happens in the stomach alone is an extremely complicated symphony of reactions. This could possibly be why gastroparesis takes on so many different manifestations and why responses are so variable for each person.

The following paragraphs are important to begin to understand what should be happening in your stomach. But, if you don't want to get into the science of it, feel free to skim. The science is certainly fascinating, however, and by skimming it, I hope you get the immense complexity of how the stomach works, and how there are a variety of things that could possibly be malfunctioning to cause the symptoms you are having.

What makes the stomach work is a fantastically coordinated effort between your nervous system, the secretions within your stomach walls, and smooth muscle cells. I'll go through the different pieces, which can all be broken down into smaller parts and their functions, and provide a better idea of how complicated it can be.

ANATOMY OF THE STOMACH

The stomach itself is broken down into four main parts: the cardiac region, the fundus, the corpus, and the pylorus.

CARDIAC REGION: Food comes to the cardiac region directly after it's been swallowed through the esophagus. This part of the stomach secretes an alkaline mucus, so if any food should come back up through the esophagus, there is a small measure of protection for your esophagus in case of acid reflux.

FUNDUS AND CORPUS: These two regions function together, and along with the cardiac region, they are referred to as the *proximal stomach*. This is the area of the stomach where most of your storage takes place, and is why, when it is working correctly, you can get away with having a few meals a day. The lining of the fundus and corpus includes glands that release pepsinogen (a precursor to the enzyme pepsin, which breaks down proteins), and stomach acid. The glands in these regions also produce a mucus that safeguards the lining of the stomach from the acid it produces. Another important secretion of the fundus and corpus is called intrinsic factor. Intrinsic factor is necessary for the absorption of vitamin B12, which I'll discuss more in depth on page 71.

The smooth muscle contractions of this upper part of the stomach are generally more relaxed in terms of muscle contractions, compared to the lower part.

PYLORUS: This portion of the stomach is called the *distal stomach*. The pylorus can also be broken up into two sections: the pyloric antrum, which connects to the body of the stomach, and the pyloric canal, which opens into the duodenum (small intestine). This is where the bulk of digestion happens, because this is where enzymes are secreted and more contractions take place. The distal stomach has a strong muscular wall, so ideally, the contractions should mechanically turn the food into chyme, a soupy mixture of food that is mixed with enzymes and stomach acid.

When it is stretched with food, the pyloric antrum also secretes gastrin, a hormone that stimulates acid production and motility.

The distal part of the stomach also has the job of slowly releasing chyme into the first part of small intestine. This first part of the small intestine can only manage a small bit of chyme at a time, so the small intestine releases a hormone called secretin that slows down the motility of the stomach.

The figure below helps to give a better overview of the different parts of the stomach.

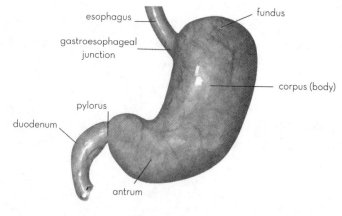

The Stomach

DUODENUM: The duodenum isn't actually part of the stomach; it's the first part of the small intestine. However, it reacts to the stomach, so it's an important piece of the puzzle.

The duodenum secretes some important hormones. When the first bit of acid from the first drop of chyme reaches the duodenum, the hormone secretin is released. Secretin has two major functions: to stimulate the pancreas to release bicarbonate, which will neutralize the acid in the small intestine; and to slow down stomach activity, as mentioned above.

The second important hormone that the duodenum secretes is called *cholecystokinin (CCK)*. This hormone stimulates the release of bile from the gallbladder and is vital in helping to digest fats.

From the previous figure, we can see where each part of the stomach is located. The explanations above give us simple descriptions of their actions. Isolated, these are just interesting facts. But it is also useful to understand that all of these actions are in essence *reactions* to chemical signaling from one part of the stomach to another. Remember, this is the enteric nervous system working on its own.

Here are some interesting reactive events:

- The vagus nerve (which, remember, is a cranial nerve with motor and sensory fibers that pass from the brain stem through multiple organs) stimulates the release of acetylcholine, a neurotransmitter that stimulates the release of stomach acid in the stomach.

- When the stomach begins to expand, stretch receptors in the antrum release gastrin, a hormone that tells the parietal cells in the fundus to release stomach acid.

- When the pylorus senses that there is acidic chyme in the lower part of the stomach, it releases somatostatin, which is another hormone that slows down stomach motility.

- The parietal cells release pepsinogen, which is the precursor to pepsin, the enzyme that breaks down proteins into amino acids. Pepsinogen only converts into pepsin when it comes into contact with stomach acid! Makes sense, right? That way, it doesn't start working on the body's own proteins; it only activates when it hits the inside of the stomach.

THE IMPORTANCE OF STOMACH ACID

Something that isn't adequately looked at in digestion is the importance of stomach acid. Stomach acid can sound harsh. When you think about having heartburn or ulcers, the idea of stomach acid comes up, and it can intuitively feel like you should have less, not more.

I'm a big believer in intuition, but this is one place where it doesn't serve. You need adequate stomach acid. It helps you to break apart proteins, absorb minerals, and break down your food. You also need adequate stomach acid to absorb vitamin B12. One theory behind GERD and acid reflux is that there is too little stomach acid, and food will then start to ferment in the stomach and create air pockets that push food back up the esophagus. Plus, everything in the digestive system is cause and effect. If there is not enough stomach acid mixing with your food, then certain hormones that are involved along the complicated chain may not be released.

As a nutrition coach, I have had people come to me with digestive problems (bloating, horrible gas) that were fixed by simply supporting their acid production.

Far too often, acid reducers like proton pump inhibitors (PPI) are prescribed for stomachaches. The proton pump is responsible for acid production. One study looked at a university teaching hospital and how they prescribed proton pump inhibitors. According to the study, "PPI prescribing rates among inpatients are high, and frequently not evidence based."[16] I, myself, am an example of someone who had severe stomachaches all through childhood, and all I was ever given were acid reducers. It wasn't until my late twenties that a doctor figured out I had an *H. pylori* infection and gave me the right kind of treatment to deal with the infection. I'm now stomachache free.

When people take acid reducers for too long, stomach acid can be reduced to a point that's detrimental to health and to digestion. Remember that you *need* acid to digest your food and absorb adequately.

So, acid production is important. (Refer to Appendix B to increase stomach acid holistically.)

It's impossible to talk about acid production and not about the importance of hormones and how they affect acid production and digestion. We've already named a few hormones: CCK, secretin, and somatostatin, and there are many that specifically affect acid production, such as gastrin. There are, however, many more that either enhance or slow down motility in different parts of the digestive system, and signal other parts of the digestive system to work. It's quite dizzying, actually. I don't think you need to study and learn every single hormone and what it does. You do need to walk away from this section realizing what a complicated and incredible symphony your digestive system is.

Another thing to note is that even if you are getting most of your nutrition from formula or are using a feeding tube most of the time, it is useful to find out what foods still work for you so that you can practice using your digestive system. Swallowing is important, and simply having food in your stomach is important, because all of these things will signal the digestive system to do things, and our body in its entirety follows a use-it-or-lose-it framework.

---

16 C. Owen, et al., "PTU-001 Overuse of Proton Pump Inhibitors and Strategies to Reduce Inappropriate Prescribing," *Gut* (2014), DOI: 10.1136/gutjnl-2014-307263.75.

ENZYMES

Enzymes also deserve special mention because there are thousands of enzymes that work in your digestive system to create chain reactions and help break down different categories of food. An enzyme is a substance that acts as a catalyst (it starts the process) for a biological process. Whenever you hear of something in the body that ends with -ase, it refers to an enzyme. It's no surprise that they only work in certain environments and conditions, providing yet another reminder of how when one thing is off, then it can throw everything off. One enzyme I've already touched on, pepsin, is produced in the stomach and initiates the breakdown of proteins into smaller components.[17] Pepsin requires an acidic environment to do its work, another nod to the importance of stomach acid.

There are digestive enzymes that you can take over the counter, and they can be extremely helpful in aiding digestion, but I would do this with the advice of a naturopathic doctor or holistic nutritionist. It's never a good idea to simply start taking supplements because you hear that it has helped someone.

Personal Insight
Allie, 34, Colorado

When were you diagnosed with gastroparesis?
September 2015.

Tell us your diagnosis story.
It all started about two years ago. I had been having symptoms (vomiting and feeling nauseous) for a while and was misdiagnosed with gallbladder and appendix problems.

One time, things became severe enough that I was hospitalized. It was bizarre; I remember eating a really big turkey sandwich, something that I would normally never eat, and I remember feeling really full and uncomfortable that evening.

---

17 Michael Gershon, *The Second Brain*, (New York: Harper Collins, 1998).

I woke up and started vomiting over and over again for the next two days. My stomach was distended, and it felt super strange—it was like I had the stomach flu, but much more violent. I finally went to the doctor. My white blood cell count was really high. They thought I had an intestinal blockage, prepared me for surgery, went in, and found a mesenteric hematoma[18] on the abdominal wall. My doctor now thinks it was caused by my excessive vomiting.

I was hospitalized because I couldn't keep anything down. They put a tube into my stomach to suck up everything and then they discharged me. Afterward, I could ingest little things, like liquid and oatmeal. At this point, I wasn't diagnosed yet. I consumed a lot of protein drinks at the time. The other problem was that I didn't have an appetite. I didn't think about eating food, but I slowly moved into a regular diet over time.

Then I had knee surgery later that year. I was on pain medication, and I was symptomatic again. I wasn't able to tolerate alcohol, although I was still able to tolerate normal foods. Since then, it's been a gradual shift, and my diet has gotten more and more narrow.

When I finally got diagnosed, I did a gastric emptying test. I ate a radioactive egg and the test took scans of my stomach to see where the egg was in the digestive system. Mine came back as a severe case of having slow digestion. However, I'm not the worst-case scenario in my symptoms, even though they are bad, and I'm able to keep up a healthy weight.

I'm now in the phase where I'm trying new things within the realm of gastroparesis-friendly foods, and I just want to get out of a rut. I'm trying to eat what a normal meal would be with other people. I've found it to be really isolating, because I was on a sausage-puree diet for eight months. I'm just starting to break free from that. What works for me is to

---

18 A mesenteric hematoma is localized bleeding in the bowel.

have two meals a day of soft, liquid-pureed foods. My dinner meal is more normal and can be a more social meal.

Did the conventional diet wisdom of low fat, low fiber work for you?

I feel like the fiber part is true for me. I'm able to tolerate dairy. Sometimes I need dairy for protein. I am able to tolerate coconut oil, butter, and full-fat dairy. I can have avocado; salmon is OK. I cannot have nut butter. I don't know if it's the nuts.

Which foods don't work for you?

Beans are terrible, because of the fiber, and so is chunky vegetable soup. Any hard meats, salads, fresh fruit, apples, spicy things. My taste buds now like things that are really bland. Nothing with citrus, no oranges, limes...it just doesn't taste good. Broccoli... Green beans... The sad thing is that I just want to eat a salad, but I just can't.

What foods work well for you?

Pureed squash, sweet potatoes, any kind of blended soups. Sautéed spinach works well, watermelon, bananas, avocados. Light fish works well, ground meat works fine, and I'm gluten free now. When I do eat gluten, I feel a little more symptomatic; sometimes I have gluten-free pasta. Recently, I've been able to eat gluten-free pizza with a little bit of tomatoes. Just a little bit.

I don't weigh anything out, I just eyeball the amount. For me, it's about two handfuls. I haven't really converted to eating six small meals a day. I have a hard time meal planning and remembering to eat. I don't feel hungry. I feel almost better when I don't eat.

Have complementary therapies worked for you?

Acupuncture. I go to acupuncture once a week, and sometimes twice a week if I'm having a really bad week.

Also, I really think that seeing a therapist has helped a lot, even though it took me a while to jump on this train. The more that I'm learning about it, the more I see that the mind/body connection is so strong. I find that a reduction of stress at any level reduces my symptoms. Seeing a therapist has helped me stop destructive patterns. For example, I would wake up feeling sick, and then I would vomit right away, or I would just feel really nauseous and vomit. I would think, "Oh my gosh, what did I do? I don't have time for this." Sometimes your mind can just go crazy. Sometimes the stomach isn't working right that day, and I would get all flustered about it. I was calling in sick at least once a pay period. It just got to the point that it was really hard to deal with in a day-to-day way. Now, after seeing a therapist, my mental process is not about freaking out and making it worse. I just say, "It's ok, because the times I'm getting sick are lesser, and I'm able to rebound quicker. I can get sick and even go to work."

Have you discovered any tricks that help you to feel better?
I wear antinausea wristbands for motion sickness. It's an acupressure point for nausea. Laying still and closing my eyes will help with the nausea...that has definitely helped.

I don't get massages regularly, but those have helped. Abdominal massage. That seems to feel good, and get things moving.

I just started trying to do yoga. I feel like it's helping. I'm still trying to figure out the right balance of physical activity.

What advice would you give to someone newly diagnosed?
Be patient, because that's been the hardest struggle. It feels like it takes a long time before you start to see small changes of relieving symptoms.

What I find interesting about Allie's story is that her second bout of symptoms coincided with taking pain medications. This may or may not have been the case, but nonsteroidal anti-inflammatory drugs, or NSAIDs, while stopping pain, can also stop the healing of the stomach lining and affect blood flow and other functions of mucosal lining. Without proper mucosal lining, the walls of the stomach are vulnerable to stomach acid.[19] While gastroparesis isn't necessarily about the halting of mucosal secretions, these drugs do affect functions in the stomach. If we follow the idea that one thing can throw off everything else, this can be an important aspect to consider. This is just another thing to think about when taking too many medications—there are always side effects.

❧

The stomach, along with the entire digestive system, is a complicated beast. There are many places that it can be hindered. However, the human body is an incredible piece of machinery, and new connections are being made all the time. Your resilient body can adapt to pretty much anything.

Michael D. Gershon, in his informative book *The Second Brain*, shares some positive words. As he outlines the digestive system, he does say that we can live without the functions of the stomach. Quality of life is decreased, but we can make do. He says that the loss of storage (which means that we have to eat more meals a day) is more bothersome than the loss of its digestive capabilities. Our small intestine can make do without it. He also says that it's the intrinsic factor that we can't live without, so again, refer to page 71, where we talk about vitamin B12 supplementation.

This is positive news, however bothersome it may be. We can learn to manage life with gastroparesis, and learn to manage it well.

---

19 D. Fromm, "How Do Non-steroidal Anti-inflammatory Drugs Affect Gastric Mucosal Defenses?" *Clinic Investment Medicine* 10, no. 3 (May 1987), http://www.ncbi.nlm.nih.gov/pubmed/3304754.

Chapter 3
CREATING A HOLISTIC PLAN FOR GASTROPARESIS

Being healthy, feeling good, feeling strong. However you say it, it's an elusive goal for everyone. Not to mention that each of us will define this in a different way. Feeling healthy for you will be different from feeling healthy for me, or feeling healthy for my mother, or feeling healthy for the cancer patient.

I recently took a movement and alignment course with an incredibly intelligent woman named Judith Aston, who created a way of looking at the body that she calls the Aston Paradigm. A basic tenet in her philosophy is about finding your available neutral. Judith describes neutral as the "position that creates the least stress and the most support for your body."[20]

---

20 Judith Aston, *Moving Beyond Posture*, (USA: Amazon, 2007)

Judith also says that "finding neutral is about honoring who you are at any given time."[21] This is an important idea for all of us.

I love the idea about your best available neutral, since it is much like this moving target of health. It's about honoring how you are feeling on that day and making sure you are making the best decision to honor where you are. When I was conducting interviews with GP folks, sometimes someone was going through a flare-up and had to reschedule. And that is something that might be a part of your daily life moving forward. Your body, some days, will not allow you to keep a set schedule of appointments. I admired the boundaries that people had, knowing their own bodies and how to make a decision that was best for their physical and mental health.

There are days that you will undoubtedly feel frustrated, maybe angry, maybe on the edge of despair. How do you honor that, acknowledge that, and then also take actions to find your best available neutral?

You are most likely feeling overwhelmed, and that's completely normal. Remember, though, that you are not alone, and to be compassionate with yourself. There's no rush to an end goal. You are just here to take it step by step as you figure out what works for your body and what doesn't.

This is where we'll start to create a plan to give you some structure with which to take action. Only take what resonates with you, and leave the rest.

I'll first talk about your supporting protocol. I am grateful for an interview I did with Crystal Saltrelli, who is also an author and health coach that works with GPers. She said something that I think is really important: "Your food did not cause your gastroparesis." Essentially, she feels that there is too much emphasis placed on the

---

21 Ibid.

diet. I interpret this to mean that something happened in your life or in your health that may have made you more susceptible to falling ill. This is a better time than any to think about what that event or environment could have been. How were you taking care of yourself when GP first started, and what are some changes you can make for the better now? I'll help you think about things, and if you make a change, who knows? If it's a change for the better, then something positive will always come out of it.

In this chapter, we look at the foundational piece of your lifestyle in three sections:

1. Lifestyle Assessment: Here, you'll take a moment to think about what's been going on in your life and find support regarding those areas.

2. Finding Medical Support: First things first, find a support team. I'll talk more about helpful players and communities that you can be a part of.

3. Reducing Stress: In this section, I'll discuss how you can create a lifestyle where even when you are having severe flare-ups, you can find support and some serenity. In order for healthy digestion to work, your body must be in a state of relaxation.

Then we'll discuss a structure for how you can find nourishing habits and foods that work for you. I'll identify some aspects of your life that you might not think are related to nourishing yourself. I'll also talk about the importance of a whole foods, non-artificial diet. Plus, it's worthwhile to talk about some categories of foods that some GPers find problematic. But again, there's not much rhyme or reason for that, and it's all about figuring out what works best for you.

LIFESTYLE ASSESSMENT

Any person can benefit from taking a look at how they live. Gastroparesis has come into your life, so what are you going to do with this change?

In this section, you'll take an assessment to start to look at areas that could be causing stress, which is an idea I'll talk about a lot in the next section.

Before I do, I'd like to focus on another idea that I find extremely interesting: sometimes, there are emotional and mental influences on certain parts of the body. Louise Hay, who wrote an interesting book called *Heal Your Body*, connects certain symptoms and physical manifestations to mindsets and emotional causes. For the stomach, in particular, she relates that the stomach is connected to the concepts of nourishment and digesting ideas, dread, fear of the new, and inability to assimilate the new.

These ideas may not ring true to you at all, but if there is something tugging at your mind, it will be interesting to think on it more, and see perhaps what effect it may have on your physical body.

Louise Hay also has some meditations online, and I found this one particularly inspiring:

"There are many things that you can do to assist in your own healing. Body, Mind and Spirit must be balanced. It sounds more overwhelming than it is. Just begin where you are, doing what you can. It's like cleaning a house, it doesn't matter what room you begin, if you keep going, eventually the whole house will be clean."[22]

I love this analogy of the house. You can start anywhere, and in fact, start where you are most inspired to start. Maybe that is your room, or your kitchen. Anywhere works. So, let's begin.

---

22 Louise Hay, "40 Minutes Every Day to Change Your Life Forever," November, 2014, Accessed August 4, 2016, https://www.youtube.com/watch?v=jbdB2ss1YLs.

HOLISTIC HEALTH QUESTIONNAIRE

Health Questions	Often	Seldom	Never
Do you eat home-cooked food?			
Do you eat organic foods?			
Do you feel like you are adequately hydrated?			
Do you eat colorful foods daily?			
Do you eat quickly and not chew thoroughly?			
Do you eat cooked and heated foods?			
Do you smoke?			
For women, are you on birth control pills?			
Do you get less than seven hours of sleep a night?			
Do you sit most of the day?			
Do you exercise?			
Do you eat foods that are in packages?			
Do you spend time doing a creative hobby or art form?			
Do you spend quality time with friends and family?			
Do you consider yourself a valuable part of your community?			
Do you practice self-care (baths, massages, treating yourself)?			
Do you spend time learning something you are interested in?			
Do you feel stressed?			

A few of these questions warrant explanation, so let's look them.

DO YOU SMOKE? Most people at least understand the dangers of smoking in terms of healthy lungs and overall health. For you, smoking, or nicotine specifically, is shown to affect and slow down gastric emptying.[23] Other studies have found that it delayed gastric emptying of solids, but liquids were not affected.[24]

Suffice it to say that there are a multitude of benefits if you decide to stop smoking, including helping increase the motility of solid foods in your stomach. It's worth thinking about quitting and looking into programs that help with smoking cessation. Hypnosis can be a powerful tool.

DO YOU TAKE BIRTH CONTROL PILLS? Many women find that their GP symptoms vary with their menstrual cycle. A woman's menstrual cycle works like this: The first day of your period is the first day of the menstrual cycle. In general, a women's menstrual cycle is 28 days, but can vary from person to person. The first 14 days are called the follicular phase, and is when the body releases estrogen. Estrogen acts to build the lining of the uterus, called the endometrium. When estrogen peaks, an egg is released. If the egg is not fertilized, the body enters the luteal phase. This is where the body begins releasing progesterone, which will cause the lining of the uterus to shed, and your period will start at the end of the 28 days. The figure below shows the rise in estrogen and then the rise in progesterone (top graphic) in relation to the thickness of the endometrium (bottom graphic). The dotted line indicates ovulation.

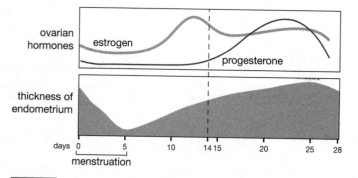

23 Gritz, et al., "The Effect of Nicotine on the Delay of Gastric Emptying," *Alimentary Pharmacology and Therapeutics* 2, no. 2 (April 1988), http://www.ncbi.nlm.nih.gov/pubmed/2979243.

24 Miller, et al., "Smoking Delays Gastric Emptying of Solids," *Gut* 30, no. 1 (January 1989), http://www.ncbi.nlm.nih.gov/pmc/articles/PMC1378230.

Women often report that their GP symptoms worsen during the luteal phase (the second half) of their menstrual cycle. This makes sense, because progesterone is known to slow down motility. This is why in pregnancy, when there is an increase in progesterone, there can be symptoms of gastrointestinal distress: nausea, vomiting, bloating, constipation. Progesterone is known to affect smooth muscle contractions, and we know from our discussion of digestion that smooth muscle is responsible for peristalsis, or motility.

If you are a woman and have never charted your menstrual cycle before, it's a very interesting exercise. There are many family planning books out there that go through the process in detail (although of course they focus on trying to get pregnant, or avoiding it...whatever may be the case), a great book being *The Garden of Fertility* by Katie Singer. In your case, however, it would be interesting to notice if there is a correlation between where you are in your menstrual cycle and your severity of symptoms.

What about birth control pills? Birth control pills are made up of different synthetic hormones, namely estrogen and progestin. Progestin is the synthetic form of progesterone.

Birth control pills are excellent at preventing pregnancy because they stop the body from releasing an egg. Plus, there have been some studies done that show those on birth control have less fluctuation in symptoms, particularly nausea and rapid fullness.[25] Nothing, however, is conclusive, simply because there haven't been that many studies done. As with anything that you hear, you have to examine and try for yourself. If you aren't trying to prevent pregnancy, looking to go on birth control to manage your symptoms might not be the best thing because they do have other side effects that are discussed often in the holistic community.

---

25 Verrengia et al., "Variation of Symptoms during the Menstrual Cycle in Female Patients with Gastroparesis," *Neurogastroenterology and Motility* 23, no. 7 (February 17, 2011). DOI: 10.1111/j.1365-2982.2011.01681.x.

Birth control pills cause certain nutrients to be depleted, and since you are in a compromised nutritional state already, it's something to think about. Birth control pills deplete folic acid, vitamins B2, B6, B12, C, and E, and the minerals magnesium, selenium, and zinc.[26] They can also affect other aspects of health, such as libido, emotions, and oxidative stress. Dr. Kelly Brogan has a great article on other possible side effects of birth control pills.[27]

Personally, the last time I got off birth control pills, I remember thinking, "Oh! This is what having emotions feels like." If you are someone acutely aware of your body, it will be an interesting experiment.

DO YOU EAT COOKED AND WARMED FOODS? The temperature of your foods could be affecting your gastric motility. Generally, the higher the temperature, the quicker the gastric emptying.[28] This is an accepted thought in Western medicine, and it makes sense as it also follows the thought lines of both traditional Chinese medicine and ayurveda.

Traditional Chinese medicine and ayurveda describe the stomach as a simmering pot and a digestive fire. When you eat foods cold and uncooked, you lower the temperature of your simmering pot, just like when you bring a pot up to a simmer and add an ingredient, you then need to wait for it to come to a boil again. Your digestion is much the same way. So according to these traditional ways of looking at nutrition, eating cooked foods and warm foods is better for your digestion.

It would be interesting to experiment on how your stomach feels when you drink a smoothie as opposed to a pureed vegetable soup.

26 M. Palmery, et al., "Oral Contraceptives and Changes in Nutritional Requirements," *European Review for Medical and Pharmacological Sciences* 17, no. 13 (July 2013), http://www.ncbi.nlm.nih.gov/pubmed/23852908.

27 Kelly Brogan, MD, "That Naughty Little Pill. Birth Control Side Effects," Mad in America (February 8, 2013), Accessed September 1, 2016, https://www.madinamerica.com/2013/02/that-naughty-little-pill.

28 David Boomer, "Gastrointestinal Physiology," last modified November 28, 2015, Accessed August 2, 2016, https://www.boomer.org/c/p3/c22/c2203.html.

Mindset Questions	Often	Seldom	Never
Do you have things that you look forward to each day?			
Do you use the word "can't" or "never"?			
Do you feel like you have a purpose to fulfill in your life?			
Do you love yourself?			
Do you say mean things to yourself?			
Do you often wish things were different?			
Do you laugh?			
Do you feel like you sacrifice in your life?			
Do you take risks?			

What is your mindset? Some of the mindset questions are there specifically to challenge the language that you use to talk to yourself. My former self believed that language wasn't a big deal, that I didn't really mean things that I said. Now, though, I see how powerful language is, even small changes in the words we use. What we tell ourselves is extremely important. The little voice inside your head can make or break you, and the sooner you start to understand what it habitually says, the more control you have to make it say something different. Again, take this questionnaire as information, and use it to begin to observe your own thoughts and mindset.

Let's look back at the questionnaire. Regardless of what you answered, this is feedback for you. These are by no means all of the questions that could be asked, nor are they judgments. If a question brings some feelings up, that's informative. No one else knows why this is so, except for you.

Make a note of what areas are growing edges for you. Keep a list of areas that you'd like to work on. Do you keep a journal? A video diary? I have found that writing is a very cathartic process, and when I write in my journal, I'm actually writing to myself. It's a place that I can be real and honest. It's where I can get my feelings out. If you keep one already, perhaps you know what I'm talking about. Every once in a while, I make lists of things I'd like to work on or mindsets I'd like to change. Ultimately, it's a place where I can share things, and put them out into the world, and also revisit. There's no better record of growth and change than your own words from years before. Think about starting one.

Personal Insight
Crystal Saltrelli, 32, New York

When were you diagnosed with GP?
In 2004.

What is your diagnosis story?
I initially thought I had asthma and went to see the pulmon-ologist. He thought my issues were actually gastrointestinal issues. So I went to a gastroenterologist, and they treated me for acid reflux with a proton pump inhibitor. I was having a lot of nausea, instant fullness, and reflux. I didn't realize I had GP symptoms until I read the symptoms. I would eat three bites and be full after being starving. After about a year, I went to see another GI doctor. He did a gastric emptying test. I didn't know what he was testing for, I just knew I had this test. When I went for the follow up, he said I had delayed emptying, I got a handout, and was told to "see what happens in three months."

In your book you mention you have a gastric stimulator, do you still have one?
Yes, I have one, but we are about to turn it off, actually. I had a gastric emptying test last April, and it came out really well. I emptied 99 percent of my stomach's contents within four hours. It's pretty huge. I have had eight or nine scans since 2004, and they have never been close to normal. I still have

other GI symptoms, but the GP symptoms have been getting increasingly better. I still have quite a limited diet.

My doctor was not surprised at my results, but I was very surprised. I had been told many times over the years that it was incurable, and it will never go away. I have had so many clients that have gotten better, but I still had trouble believing that I could also get better.

Why do you think you've gotten better?

There is no one thing that I can point to. There are a couple of things that happened in my life. I'm really into a comprehensive approach. All of that helped. I had a baby... My symptoms got better when I was pregnant, and then worsened again after. Maybe the pregnancy helped. At the same time, I had a lot of postpartum anxiety, and then I got *very* into the mind-body connection, primarily to address the anxiety, but I noticed my GI symptoms improving.

Have alternative therapies worked for you?

I have literally tried everything under the sun. From homeopathy to acupuncture, reiki, and cranial sacral... Clinical hypnosis was the most helpful for me. For me, acupuncture was more helpful for lower GI issues, like constipation. Really, it was a lot more of the self-care kind of things that helped the most, like yoga and meditation.

What tricks work for you when you are having a flare?

Honestly, for me, it seems counterintuitive; the less I tried to do, the more quickly it would get better. I would get super freaked out, "I have to take care of this now." I would try to do all these different things, meds, maybe try this thing. The combo of stress and throwing so many different things at the body was not helpful.

Relax into the flare-up. It's temporary, it has happened however many times, it will go away.

What have you learned from working with many people that have GP?

One of the things I've learned from watching other people is that we tend to have a lot more control over how we feel than we think we do. I have clients come to me who say it doesn't matter what I eat or do, I am sick all the time. Then, ultimately, after we work through nutrition/lifestyle/stress management, people say, I didn't know I had this much control.

We think this is something that happens to us; this is the message that we've been given from the medical community. They say there's nothing we can do besides take meds.

People are surprised, not that their GP is cured, but that they feel significantly better just making small changes. It is a complicated condition. It seems too big for little things to make a difference, but it's small changes that really can make a big difference.

What advice would you give someone newly diagnosed?

Putting together a plan that puts diet/lifestyle/complementary treatments with appropriate medical treatment will give someone a proper foundation to move forward. This gives you the best shot to maintaining symptoms and improving quality of life.

I think this is really important. I was chasing the diet and drugs approach. My diet was nothing more than applesauce and fruit loops. If that's what you are doing, you are only going to get sicker.

I think people focus so much on the diet, and the diet is really only one piece of the puzzle. When it comes to nutrition, your diet is the only way to get nutrition. When it comes to managing GP, nutrition is only one piece. Focusing on food as a cure for GP doesn't really work. It's important, but it's just a piece of the puzzle.

You can find learn more about Crystal Saltrelli and her work with GP folks on her website: Livingwithgastroparesis.com.

FINDING MEDICAL SUPPORT

Finding support is imperative to managing gastroparesis. There are times when you will feel very alone with your symptoms. It can be extremely isolating. Often, family members are sympathetic, but they aren't fully able to understand. In my interviews and as part of online forums, I discovered that two related pieces of advice surfaced over and over again: One, find support with an experienced medical care team and two, find a supportive community. I'll first talk about some tips to find a medical care team. (Thank you to all my interviewees, who guided in putting this list together.)

TIPS TO LOOKING FOR YOUR MEDICAL TEAM

1. Find a doctor, either a general practitioner or a gastroenterologist, that is familiar with gastroparesis. Gastroparesis is still a largely unknown condition, and it's important to work with someone who has some experience with motility issues. Crystal Saltrelli has compiled a PDF of recommendations by other GPers that could be helpful. You'll find the link in Resources on page 167.

2. Look for a doctor who is willing to admit they don't know everything. Gastroparesis is still being researched and much is not known about it. It's important to find someone who is not afraid to say they don't know something. They also shouldn't tell you that they know exactly what will happen. GP is so individual, and everybody responds to it differently.

3. Find someone you feel comfortable with. It's important to share your symptoms fully and honestly with your doctor so they know exactly what your experience is. If you don't feel comfortable sharing, perhaps you should find someone that you do feel comfortable with.

4. The right and knowledgeable doctor should be able to explain all the pros and cons to you about different medications and different surgeries. They shouldn't rush you into any particular treatment until you understand it from all angles.

5. Look for someone who also is willing to be in communication in between appointments, because you will most likely need support during those times as well. Being able to email and ask questions is helpful.

Part of your medical care team can be specialists in complementary therapy treatments, like the following:

ACUPUNCTURE: Acupuncture is a facet of traditional Chinese medicine that is becoming more and more popular in the United States. It essentially runs on the theory that we have energy meridians throughout our bodies that align with different parts of the body. Acupuncture uses small, thin needles to puncture specific points along these meridians to alleviate pain, improve circulation, and do many other things.

Many GPers find acupuncture to be helpful with pain symptoms, and many advise that consistency is key.

I myself go to acupuncture regularly, and I find that the ritual of the sessions is also very helpful to reduce stress and to slow down. I always request the point in the third eye, as it creates a sense of calm instantly. Try it!

PSYCHOTHERAPY OR PSYCHOLOGY: In my interviews, many GPers suggested seeking a therapist who works with those who have chronic illnesses. This piece is especially important because of what the mind can do to your stress levels. The mind-body connection is real and powerful because, ultimately, you have control over your thoughts. Stress is often a mindset, and it's one of the main things that can exacerbate your GP symptoms. To find support, ask for referrals from the GP community. Take Yelp reviews with a grain of salt and be open to putting some tools in your pocket that could help you cope on really hard days.

ABDOMINAL MASSAGE: With anything that is more hands on, it's important to properly vet your practitioner. Not all practitioners know what GP and its side effects are, so before seeking this possibility out, it is extremely important to consult your doctor and speak with the practitioner beforehand. Among interviewees and support group participants, some have found that abdominal massage was helpful in supporting motility. One of the possible modalities to look into is called visceral manipulation. The word *viscera* refers to internal organs, while *manipulation* means skillfully using the hands to change the current state. Some GPers have found that with this technique, their movement is better and that it is helpful to release gas. One thing you can ask the practitioner about is self-abdominal massage. If it does not cause too much pain, this could be part of a self-care practice. Another modality is called Chi Nei Tsang, which can also be helpful.

FIND A COMMUNITY

While you seek your medical dream team, which is sometimes not easy, it can really be helpful to be able to go to your community and ask for help. Your immediate community consists of your family and friends, even though you will have to educate your friends and family about this disease.

While those in your community may not understand exactly what you are going through, it's helpful to let them know what ways they can help. If you are someone who has never asked for help, sometimes this can be daunting. But providing those close to you with a few resources to learn about GP (see Resources on page 167) and a list of things that they can do to best support you is helpful.

HELPFUL TIPS ABOUT ONLINE SUPPORT

Tabatha, 35, is a GPer who, despite dealing with other medical issues along with the GP, finds fulfillment in helping others where she can, including in advocating for H.R. 2311, a functional gastric and motility act that raises awareness for funding and research for better medications. She says this about the following organizations:

"G-Pact is a wonderful organization run by volunteers who have gastroparesis. Any money they get goes into research. There are a lot of resources on their website. You can fill out a survey on their website and it goes toward collecting accurate data. On their website, you can see what other people are going through. They also send you material that can help explain the disease to friends and family members. One really helpful thing they send out is accessibility cards that can allow you to bring your own food into restaurants or get into a restroom if there's an emergency.

They have a pen pal program that I am a part of if I'm feeling down, and they will send out care packages if they know that you are in the hospital.

Association of Gastrointestinal Motility Disorders (AGMD) is also a great organization. I sit in on their monthly meetings, which you can sit in on through your computer.

Another good resource is the Oley Foundation. They have a support group and support forums. If you can't afford formula or tube feedings, they will send out info and support to get donated food. They have a great forum where you can give or sell things that you have left over, like leftover formula, for example. You can get supplies that way. If a loved one has passed away, their family members can also post supplies there."

Thanks, Tabatha, for your suggestions!

It's important to know that you are not alone with your gastroparesis. GP affects thousands and thousands of people, and awareness of the condition is becoming more widespread. Those who are first diagnosed may have never heard of this condition, and it can be daunting and overwhelming. However, there are many support groups online that are full of people who are going through very similar experiences. These forums are extremely helpful for venting when you need to, but also for asking advice about certain medications, surgeries, or cooking tips. Keep in mind that postings are often made when people are feeling at their worst, and not their best. Sometimes the overall picture you glean from online support groups can be bleaker than reality.

If you aren't in any support groups, I highly encourage you to check out the list of support groups in Resources. You don't have to post if you don't want to; simply reading and observing the community at first can be helpful.

REDUCING STRESS

In the last section, I discussed finding support, which is one of the main facets of stress reduction. In his wonderful book, *Why Zebras Don't Get Ulcers*, Robert Sapolsky refers to psychologist Shelly Taylor, who discusses the different ways that men and women deal with stress. For men, fight-or-flight is a better description, while women, the majority of GPers, are more likely to "tend and befriend" when dealing with stress.[29]

You already know that stress puts the body in sympathetic mode, which, in turn, effectively shuts down your digestion. Controlling stress, however, is easy to say, but hard to do, especially when dealing with a chronic condition. GP is an ever-fluctuating condition that can be stable for a while and then, without warning, come on strongly or change suddenly. The state at which your body is on a day-to-day, or even minute-to-minute, basis can be stressful, and accepting wherever you are at is a work in progress for many GPers. Let's look

---

29 Robert M. Sapolsky, *Why Zebras Don't Get Ulcers*, (New York: St. Martin's Griffin, 2004).

at some ways in which you can start shaping your environment. Here are some tips for when flare-ups occur.

SHAVING DOWN YOUR RESPONSIBILITIES

Depending on the severity of your gastroparesis, it may be hard to keep up with responsibilities. Missing work and letting go of appointments can be a common occurrence when flare-ups happen. Understanding what is reasonable to expect from your body is an ever-changing target, but it's helpful to look at what responsibilities you can shave off.

For parents, the guilt and stress of not being able to be the parent that they'd like to be, and also seeing how their illness affects their children and family members, can be stressful. Gastroparesis is an emotional disease for all involved, and finding support outside of the family, such as therapy for caregivers and children, might be a good option to look into.

MEDITATION

Meditation is a practice of watching your thoughts and concentrating on a specific thing. I am still working on my own mini-meditation practice, and I find it helpful to take myself away from my own thoughts and body to connect to something larger than myself. Whatever your religious or spiritual beliefs may be, meditating can be a way to tap into a higher power or energy.

Studied quite comprehensively, meditation is one of the few tools to show a positive effect on the mental health of those dealing with a chronic disease.[30] One study looked at 51 patients with different types of chronic pain. The patients went through a 10-week meditation course, practicing a method of "detached observation." There

30 Paul Grossman, et al., "Mindfulness-Based Stress Reduction and Health Benefits," *Journal of Psychosomatic Research* 57, no. 1 (July 2004), DOI: 10.1016/S0022-399(03)00573-7.

were significant reductions in the pain levels reported, and in follow-ups, there were still positive effects.[31]

If you are looking to learn more about meditation, where's a good place to start? There are many different modalities to begin with. When I first started, a yoga and spiritual teacher, Broderick Rodell (www.broderickrodell.com) suggested that I sit in a comfortable position and practice counting backwards from 50. If you lose count, just start again. He also suggested that I focus on taking five breaths, with longer exhales than inhales. Even a couple of minutes a day can be helpful.

Broderick shared his thoughts about meditation and chronic pain with me:

> *"A meditation practice can support someone in managing their pain. You don't necessarily want to detach in the sense of pretending that it is not there. Neither do you want to wallow in it. This is where mindfulness/meditation practice helps. You accept what is and work with it with equanimity. At least, this is what you work toward. Also, the benefits of tempering the stress response through meditation may help dampen pain manifestation."*

Remember, meditation is just one of the tools you can begin to employ as part of your holistic GP protocol.

If you'd like to take a class or find outside resources, there are many centers, smart phone apps, and videos out there that can teach mindfulness and simple meditation practices. The Internet can help you find centers close to you. Often, hospitals or community centers can offer meditation classes as well. Here are a few techniques I have gathered throughout my time as a health coach:

---

31 Jon Kabat-Zinn, "An Outpatient Program in Behavioral Medicine for Chronic Pain Patients Based on the Practice of Mindfulness Meditation," *General Hospital Psychiatry Journal* 4, no. 1 (April 1982), DOI: 10.1016/0163-8343(82)90026-3.

BINAURAL BEATS. I often recommend listening to binaural beats when you need some assistance coming into a relaxed state. The idea is to use certain frequencies of music to help you enter into a meditative state. You listen to binaural beats with headphones (even simple headphones that come with your smart phone work), and one frequency goes in one ear (e.g., 205 Hz), and another frequency goes in the other (e.g., 210 Hz). Your brain will create a frequency of the difference of those two different frequencies. Using the numbers of 205 Hz and 210 Hz, your brain would interpret the sounds as one 5 Hz frequency.[32] One study found that listening to binaural beats before surgery helped significantly decrease anxiety.[33]

It's a really wild phenomenon, dating back to when traditional societies used music and rhythmic beats for healing ceremonies. I am listening to binaural beats right now as I write this; I find that it helps me focus and tune out other thoughts.

There are plenty of free examples of binaural beats online. You can also find them through public music streamers, like Spotify or YouTube.

MANTRAS. Thoughts are extremely powerful. I like to think of each thought as a neural pathway, a connection in the brain that can either be a strong, deep, well-worn path, or a light sliver of a connection. The more we think a certain thought, the more well-worn that path will be.

Mantras, those few sentences that you can say over and over again, help to strengthen the thoughts that you want to have more of. It could consist of a few thoughts of gratitude, especially on days when your body does not seem to be working for you and finding gratitude or positivity are not so easy. Whether you say, "My body is strong and will work through this," or "My breath will get me through this," it

---

32 "About Binaural Beats Meditation," Binaural Beats Meditation, accessed August 31, 2016, https://www.binauralbeatsmeditation.com/the-science.

33 Padmanabhan et al., "A Prospective, Randomised, Controlled Study Examining Binaural Beat Audio and Pre-operative Anxiety in Patients Undergoing General Anaesthesia for Day Case Surgery," *Anaesthesia* 60, no. 9 (2005). DOI: 10.1111/j.1365-2044.2005.04287.x.

will help. Again, this can be part of your protocol when dealing with a flare-up.

TOTAL LOAD

An important concept to discuss when we talk about stress is *total load*. In this conversation, I will also look at all the different things that the body considers to be a stressor. Our bodies are designed to withstand and even thrive on a certain amount of stress—there is a perfect balance. The concept of total load can be thought of as a bucket that can tip when it gets too full. Things that can fill this bucket are stressors.

Stressors to the body include:

- Mental stress
- Lack of sleep
- Lack of movement
- Nutritional deficiencies
- Toxins from food and environment
- Infections

When you reach your total load, your immune system can run into trouble and become more susceptible to colds, sickness, and other ailments. I've already discussed some ways to decrease mental stress and I'll discuss nutritional deficiencies in more detail on page 55.

Lack of Sleep

Sleep is often elusive for GP patients, especially when flare-ups are happening. One of the major symptoms and experiences for GPers is fatigue, which can be coupled with an inability to sleep because of symptoms.

Sleep, especially deep sleep, is essential for repair and healing. When you are having a flare-up, the best thing to do is rest, and ideally, sleep. Any sleep is helpful, however, and the more naturally you can attain it, the better, although some GPers do find help from sleep medications.

Here are some ways to invite the healing of sleep.

MAKE YOUR BEDROOM A DARK HAVEN. Our bodies respond to the light and the dark cycles of each day, also called circadian rhythm. When your body perceives it's light out, it releases cortisol that helps you wake up. When it's dark, your body releases melatonin, which helps ease it into sleep.

For those of us who live in urban centers, light pollution is a problem. One of the simplest things you can do is to get dark shades that shut out light. I live in an urban center, and as soon as I used these, I felt a huge difference. My clients, as well, find them extremely helpful. Also, cover any blinking lights you have, or better yet, unplug them. I understand the desire to see when you get up in the middle of the night, but there are studies that show that melatonin is inhibited by light.

TAKE OUT THE ELECTRONICS. Playing on your phone or watching videos late at night can be very stimulating, making it harder to go to sleep. In *Zapped*, Ann Louise Gittleman talks about all the possible consequences from the multitude of electronics we use. Certain people are very sensitive, and they find when they remove electronics from their bedroom, they get better sleep. I personally put my cell phone on airplane mode and try to leave my computer in the living room. Although I am not a particularly sensitive person, I *feel* better about it, and that makes an intangible difference.

USE SOME LAVENDER. Dab on some lavender essential oil or body spray. In one study, lavender was shown to help increase sleep in both men and women.[34]

---

34 N. Goel, et al., "An Olfactory Stimulus Modifies Nighttime Sleep in Young Men and Women," *Chronobiology International* 22, no. 5 (2009): 889-904, DOI: 10.1080/07420520500263276.

BE MINDFUL OF YOUR CAFFEINE INTAKE THROUGHOUT THE DAY.
Caffeine has a half-life of roughly six hours, meaning that it takes six hours for caffeine to fall to one-half of its potency. It takes caffeine 12 hours to completely leave your system. Having a cup in the morning shouldn't be a problem, but later on in the afternoon, it could affect your sleep.

GET SOME EXERCISE. Exercise has been shown to improve sleep. I'll talk more about this in the next section.

TAKE A LITTLE MAGNESIUM. Magnesium is one of the few supplements with many studies to back up its effectiveness as a sleep aid.[35] Taking 200 to 400 milligrams of magnesium citrate or glycinate before bed can help relax the nervous system and muscles.

Lack of Movement

Movement can be hard to manage at times when fatigue or other symptoms are at the forefront, and depending on the severity of what is going on, at times the best thing to do is *not* move.

However, movement is healing for the mind as well as the body. Doing some gentle stretches can do wonders. Moderate exercise has been shown in studies to help with motility,[36] while strenuous exercise has been shown to decrease motility.[37] It can often be the case that a lot of will is needed to start, but invariably, afterward you will feel better. Here are some ideas of moderate exercise.

YOGA. Yoga is a mixture of breathing techniques, meditation, and movement. One nice thing about yoga is that you really can go at your own pace. It's popular enough that you can pretty much find a class anywhere, and you can even find yoga videos online that you

35 Behnood Abbasi, et al., "The Effect of Magnesium Supplementation on Primary Insomnia in Elderly: A Double-Blind Placebo-Controlled Clinical Trial," *Journal of Research Medical Sciences* 17, no. 12 (2012), http://www.ncbi.nlm.nih.gov/pmc/articles/PMC3703169.

36 Prado de Oliveira, et al., "The Impact of Physical Exercise on the Gastrointestinal Tract," *Current Opinion in Clinical Nutrition and Metabolic Care* 12, no. 533 (2009), DOI: 10.1097/MCO.0b013e32832e6776.

37 B. P. Brown et al., "Strenuous Exercise Decreases Motility and Cross-Sectional Area of Human Gastric Antrum," *Digestive Diseases and Sciences* (May 1994). DOI: 10.1007/BF02087541.

can do from your home. An interesting option is Restorative Yoga, which is a collection of movements meant to relax and restore. If you find yourself in a class, it's always a good idea to let the teacher know you'll be taking things at your own pace.

ASTON FITNESS. Judith Aston has created an interesting and simple set of loosening movements that can even be done while lying down in bed, so, at the very least, you can do some movements to help keep your joints and tissues hydrated. You can find someone certified in Aston Patterning in by visiting www.astonkinetics.com/practitioners.

TESTIMONIAL FOR MOVEMENT

Tae-Lynn, 54, outside of Philadelphia

"It's important to move, no matter what chronic illness you have. I do light stretching now. When I was in physical therapy that had a warm therapy pool that was 93 to 95 degrees, it helped all my different conditions, even if I went in with a bloated belly. After I finished, it would feel so much better."

Not all movement is created equal, however, and Tae-Lynn also mentioned that crunches exacerbate her symptoms. Tae-Lynn has many other health conditions on top of her GP. This is pretty common. Her own work involves spreading kindness, something she attributes to her ability to manage her many symptoms. Find out what works for you. You can read more about her advice on page 146.

WALKING. A short walk around your neighborhood can be something simple that you can start doing now. It can also be a great way to make a date with a friend or spouse after a meal. The message boards are full of comments about how walking after a meal is helpful for getting things down.

DO WHAT YOU EXCITES YOU. It's one thing to not feel like moving because you don't feel well, but after you start moving, you should be engaged in what you are doing. If you are constantly checking the time or afterward wish you had spent your time elsewhere, then find something else that can keep you more engaged.

Nutritional Deficiencies

The state of our food production today is pretty complicated and requires some research to fully understand what is going on. I feel comfortable saying that the type of food that is available now in the US has most definitely contributed to the many different types of digestive disorders that we have now.

I've included some resources on page 167 if you are interested in learning more about our food system, as we are only going to touch on things briefly here. Finding clean foods that work for you will put the least stress on your already-stressed system. Eating foods that are heavily processed and filled with artificial and nonorganic ingredients could be more taxing to your system in the long run.

I've often heard from GPers that they could eat processed food all day and feel fine. Sometimes, it will be necessary to rely on drinks like Ensure and other processed foods to make it through the day. Although possibly more simple to digest, the other chemicals that you absorb from the food can create greater stress on your body overall. Therefore, when you are able and have the energy and space for it, eating cleanly will have a less negative impact on your body over time. The recipes that you will find in the second half of this book emphasize simple and whole food ingredients. I also dive deeper into the importance of organic foods in Nutrition 101 on page 149.

I want to talk a bit about food storage in this section, as it goes along with the conversation of what we can control in the environment to minimize total load. What we store our food in is important for our health and for the environment.

A lot of clamor exists around something called BPA, or bisphenol phosphate A, which is a synthetic compound that has been used to make plastic since the sixties.[38] There were studies that showed chemicals leaching into food and drink, and since 2008, there has been more federal awareness of this possibility. A lot of plastic products now boast being BPA free; however, this has not completely solved the problem. A study in 2011 focused on BPA-free products from popular stores and placed them in either saltwater or alcohol to see what came out. They found that most of the 455 items tested leached chemicals, which they called "estrogen-like" chemicals.[39]

These types of chemicals are called endocrine disrupters, affecting how your endocrine system releases hormones. Hormones are *extremely* important. They are basically chemical messengers in the body, telling it what to do. We've talked a bit about how hormones affect your stomach, and in the case of plastics, these chemicals often mimic estrogen in the body.

You don't have to have a complete understanding of all hormonal activity in the body to know that if one hormone is off, then it affects the others. This is just another holistic way to look at the body. Nothing exists in isolation, especially when it comes to your health. For you, we are trying to lower the stress on the body, and the cleaner we can make the food we eat, the better.

How should your habits change? Below are some simple tips that you can follow to store food safely.

- Store food in glass. My favorite storage vessels are mason jars, which come in all sorts of different sizes, are made in the US, and can serve in both your pantry and the fridge.

- Avoid heating plastic. Keep plastic out of your microwave and out of your dishwasher.

---

38 Brent A. Bauer, "What Is BPA, and What Are the Concerns about BPA?" March 11, 2016, Accessed September 4, 2016, http://www.mayoclinic.org/healthy-lifestyle/nutrition-and-healthy-eating/expert-answers/bpa/faq-20058331.

39 Chun Z. Yang, et al., "Most Plastic Products Release Estrogenic Chemicals: A Potential Health Problem that Can Be Solved." *Environmental Health Perspectives* 119 (July 2011), DOI: 10.1289/ehp.1003220.

- Get rid of old, scratched plastic. I hate that so much plastic ends up in our landfills, but if you can't recycle it, there's not much else to do about it, except be more mindful of future plastic purchases. There is a lot of information online about the harm that plastic does to our environment. If you are interested, there is more information in the resource section.

We live in a very polluted world, much of which you can't control. Paying attention to the toxins in your environment is one of the ways that you can lighten the total load that you place on your body. I'll talk about toxins from food in the next section, but first, I'll discuss toxins that you can pull in from skin care and household products.

The skin is extremely absorbent, and one way to introduce toxins into the body is through your skin care products. There are a lot of numbers out there on how many beauty products people use, but from what I can observe through friends and family, even those who are pretty minimalist use one or two on a daily basis.

Have you looked at the ingredients label on your shampoo or lotion? The FDA doesn't regulate what goes into beauty products, so there is very little oversight over what we are actually using. A great resource is the Environmental Working Group's (EWG) Skin Deep Database. They rate many products that you normally see in the grocery store, and they have a downloadable app that you can use when you are at the store.

I personally have started making my own dry shampoo from arrowroot powder, and only use coconut oil on my skin. I find that I love the smell, and it absorbs really well. A good rule of thumb is not to put anything on your skin that you wouldn't eat!

The EWG also has a database of house cleaners, and a common brand like Formula 409 gets an F rating. According to the EWG, the main ingredient in Formula 409, ethanolamine, creates moderate concern for respiratory conditions! No, thank you. An old but great method for cleaning your countertops is to use one part water to one part white vinegar. Put it in a spray bottle, and you're done.

Thinking about replacing everything at once can be overwhelming, and you might be slightly attached to a product that you are using. I get it—my mother used Oil of Olay, so I had this wonderful attachment to that smell. But after looking at the ingredients with new eyes and beginning to explore simpler alternatives, there was no going back. In reality, it's about paring down, and I have saved a lot of money in the process. Think about changing things one at a time, and remember, this is about lessening the amount of stress that is placed on your body.

Infections

Infections can be frustrating, because they are out of your control. Whether it's a stomach bug or something else, infections take much of your precious energy to get rid of. Many GPers often cite an infection to be the event that started many of their symptoms.

There isn't a whole lot that you can do about infections, but the importance of talking about them in respect to total load is that if everything else is being taken care of (e.g., you are getting adequate sleep, you are getting adequate nutrition, and there are minimal stressors coming from outside sources), your body will be better equipped to handle an infection when it comes.

Personal Insight
Sam, 34, Pittsburgh

What is your diagnosis story?
I basically had to become my own doctor on how to manage and recover. It's surprising how little doctors really understand about this.

I was first diagnosed in February 2007, but it all started much, much earlier when I was a kid. My mom has said that I always had a sensitive stomach. In middle school and high school, I was getting heartburn. I went to the doctor, he put me on Prilosec (a proton pump inhibitor). I started taking it and it worked; I no longer had heartburn. I continued to blindly take Prilosec through high school, through college, and afterward. I was never told to stop taking it.

I'm an engineer by training and I'm highly analytical. I had to employ all of that to figure out the way through this maze. Fast forward to Christmas 2006. I was living in DC at the time, and I started feeling like I had a stomach bug. It didn't feel right. I began feeling queasy, and that feeling never went away. Every time I would eat, I would feel bloated and nauseous. I was having constant nausea, but I never threw up. I went to a GI doctor and went through a barrage of tests. Everything came out fine. They kept saying you are OK, there's nothing physiologically wrong with you. They diagnosed me with irritable bowel and gave me a medication called NuLev, which didn't help at all.

Through the course of a couple of months, I lost 20 to 30 pounds, which for a 185-pound man was a big difference. I didn't want to eat; I was literally starving myself. I was put on a number of other medications that didn't work. Finally, my first GI doctor said he didn't know what else to do and basically abandoned me. I researched another GI and found one, and within 10 minutes of speaking to him, he suggested a stomach emptying test. I agreed. I took the test, and that was the first definitive proof that I had delayed gastric emptying. I was digesting food, but I was digesting extremely slowly. It took my stomach four hours to empty 50 percent. This was in February 2007.

It was great to know what it finally was, but then I didn't know how to treat it. The GI doctor put me on Zelnorm, which was a drug for IBS, but it was also supposed to help with motility. As soon as I started taking the medication, it was *immediate*, immediate relief. I got my life back. Life was good and I began gaining weight, but it was short-lived. After about two months, I went to get a refill, and I learned that Zelnorm was pulled from the market. There was some marginal number that had had heart issues while taking it. I was left again in the wind, after seeing significant benefit. My doctor put me next on Reglan.

Reglan had some possible negative side effects, including involuntary motion that, if left unchecked, could be permanent. I started taking it and had some relief, but it brought on severe depression and constant fatigue. I couldn't sleep enough. I started getting the involuntary motion, and my doctor asked me to stop immediately.

I went through some other medications, including erythromycin,[40] which didn't help, and eventually that GI doctor became harder and harder to see. I found another GI doctor who was much more available to me, who brought me into his office to talk to instead of having me on the table, and who was willing to work with my medication.

With the new GI doctor, I got some domperidone from overseas, which also didn't help. Finally, I found some generic Zelnorm online, the original medication that I was taking, and again, as soon as I began taking it, I felt immediate relief. I had taken all of these medications to come back to the one that gave me relief in the first place.

Now that I had some stability in my health, I decided to look at what could possibly be causing my symptoms, and I kept coming back to the Prilosec.

During this entire time, I was still taking the Prilosec. I started looking more into stomach acid and found that it was extremely important for digestion. I was taking acid inhibitors for so long, this must have trained my stomach to stop working. I had this idea to start weaning off of Prilosec. Every time I lowered the dose, I would get some symptoms, but my stomach would eventually adjust. It took me a year to fully get off it.

---

40 Erythromycin, an antibiotic, is also known to help with motility.

Then I started pursuing getting off of Zelnorm. I started to wean myself off and my stomach would hurt a bit, then it would start to feel better.

I moved to Pittsburgh in 2011. I felt like I had regained my old life; I could eat whatever again. I was able to successfully come off of Zelnorm, but then the original issue of poor digestion came up again. Heartburn came back like crazy. My doctor warned me about the possibility of it coming back, but I thought it was better than the other symptoms I was having. I was having heartburn for about a year and a half; no matter what I ate, I would get heartburn. Eventually, I started to get stomach pain, which really freaked me out. I went to see another GI. He wanted me to start acid inhibitors again, but I knew that wasn't an option. So, in December 2013, I pursued a holistic practitioner who was a chiropractor and also worked in nutrition. In three months she overhauled my diet, got me eating whole foods, put me on supplements, and it was a total 180. She was able to improve my health more in three months than in years of seeing any of the top doctors.

In the beginning, I saw her two to three times a week. She would give me adjustments, work on my nutrition, and she also specialized in visceral manipulation, which helped to keep my digestion moving. She also suggested that I see a counselor to work through some of my stress and type-A tendencies.

I now eat an organic, whole foods diet. If I can't pronounce it, I don't eat it. If I stray from this way of eating, I get heartburn. But for now, I have never felt better.

How did you eat before?

Before I had crazy symptoms, I would eat a can of Progresso soup and think that that was healthy. I would have store-bought sandwiches that had really processed bread and lunch meat. Now I know that these things are full of chemicals, but at the time I thought I was eating healthy.

When I had my GP symptoms, I would boil and puree chicken cubes into a canned cream of mushroom soup. I never felt good after eating it, but I would be able to keep it down.

I used to drink a lot of Ensure and Enlive, two drinks that are full of chemicals, but I needed to drink them because they were highly caloric and allowed me to function.

But now, I'm eating the way that humans are supposed to eat.

What advice do you have for newly diagnosed GPers?

I'm a firm believer, because of my experience, that gastroparesis is a symptom. This is my experience with a traditional and more holistic approach. Gastroparesis is a symptom of an underlying condition. My underlying issue was my poor digestion from when I was young. GP came later, after suppressing my acid for so many years.

My suggestion to newly diagnosed is to *not lose heart*; it can be possible to heal from this. Sometimes, you may not be able to recover, but the gastroparesis is still the outcome of something else. There's something underlying it, and you have to keep looking for what's underneath. Ask yourself, what is in your diet? What is it about the way you are living? You need to pursue that. It takes time and a lot of homework and investigation. Fortunately or unfortunately, traditional and Western doctors are not equipped for this, but a holistic approach will help you get there.

Sam's story is a great illustration of working on digestion and GP symptoms holistically. He spent a lot of time finding the right medication and the right GI doctor. He looked at his tendency for type A behaviors and anxiety, worked on his diet, was patient and weaned himself off of different medications, and finally tipped the scales when he worked with a holistic practitioner. This was a *long* road, but his advice to "not lose heart" makes sense. Thanks Sam!

The previous section was all about how to reduce total load and total amount of stressors. Working on stress reduction requires a step-by-step process and a holistic way of looking at health. It's an integral part of healing and nourishing yourself, and perhaps even reading this section seemed overwhelming. Think back on which parts hit close to home, and address those first. Perhaps the sleep section got your attention, or maybe you felt that switching to an oil from a moisturizer would be easy and a simple switch. The important thing to remember is it all adds up. You may think that the lotion you use has little effect on your GP, and you are right to an extent. You are, however, looking at the cumulative effects of everything that you do. One thing at a time, one day at a time, until you are ready for the next thing.

Chapter 4
YOUR PERSONAL NUTRITION GUIDE

Finding the right medical team, building support within the community, de-cluttering your life, and thinking about decreasing total load are all important steps to holistically supporting yourself. Now is the part of the book where I talk more specifically about how to find a way to eat that can support you.

Depending on where you are in your journey, perhaps you are drinking a lot of nutritional shakes or drinks to get you through the day, or maybe you have been eating some random things and are unsure of what has been bothering you. No matter what, you are in a great place to get started. At this point, you should be eating whatever you can to get calories and nutrition. From here, though, we'll try to start adding in a cleaner way of eating, and hopefully move toward making some homemade nutritional shakes and tasty, nutrient-dense foods.

Before I get into the specifics, it's important to talk about why you want to try to eat as cleanly as possible, and why, when you can, you should focus on ingredients that come from whole, organic foods. From Sam's personal insights (page 58), I love how he discovers that the way he eats now is the way all people should be eating—with a focus on whole, organic foods.

When you eat foods that come in packages and are full of additives, you may initially feel fine, and even good, since many processed foods may not give you the same digestive issues as certain whole foods can. However, with processed foods, you are not providing yourself the nutrition you need. Processed foods wreak havoc on the body, in part because they simply don't provide the nutrients needed to thrive. Secondly, they expose your body to chemicals that it will work to get rid of, and if you remember the idea of total load, you are trying to lessen the amount of stress on your body.

On support forums and blogs, you can read what works for others and get ideas, but the most important thing to remember is that what works for them may not work for you.

The three steps to your nutrition plan are: 1. remove problem foods, 2. start to test foods and amounts (think "simple" and discover which foods and ways of eating work for you), and 3. supplementation.

1. REMOVE PROBLEM FOODS

Figuring out problem foods takes a bit of effort, and could change depending on the day. This is the beginning of really starting to get intimate with your body, and understanding and checking in with your body every day. I'm sure you've heard that one type of food is horrible for GP and another type is good, but again, every person is different, and you will find what foods work well for you. Many of the foods that are supposed to be healthy, even from a holistic nutrition standpoint, might not be appropriate for gastroparesis.

You'll be doing a somewhat modified elimination diet, which is what we use in nutrition circles to figure out food sensitivities and allergies, which are extremely common today.

A regular elimination diet usually takes out the most common allergens: wheat, corn, soy, dairy, eggs, shellfish, peanuts, tree nuts, and citrus. You might have to take out quite a bit more. Starting with broth, simple purees, and smoothies of foods that you already know work for you is what we'll focus on.

LOW FIBER

Eating low fiber is something really contrary to everything else we've been taught about eating healthy, right? Especially when you are having digestion issues that are related to slow movement, traditional advice would be to put *more* fiber in your diet. For gastroparesis sufferers, the standard protocol for gastroparesis is a low-fat and low-fiber diet. For most people that I've spoken to, low fiber holds true, while different people tend to play around a bit with the fat quantity of their meal.

In Appendix A, you'll find a list of whole foods that are low fiber; in addition, here are some tricks to help you make foods more gastroparesis-friendly and help digestion in general.

TAKE THE SKINS OFF OF FOODS. Cucumbers, potatoes, apples, and anything with skins can be hard to digest. Peel all fruits and vegetables before you cook them.

EAT COOKED FOODS. In interview after interview, I heard many people say they miss having a salad. I'm sorry to say that salads might not be anywhere in the near future for you, if ever. Raw foods are hard for average human digestion. When we cook foods, we break down cell walls that our bodies would have to break down, so in a sense, we are predigesting some of our foods. An easy, GP-friendly and nutrient-dense way to cook veggies is to steam them with a little bit of broth or water. You can steam for a longer period of time to make sure they are as soft as possible. You can then use the steaming water to make rice, or put it into a veggie soup. There are nutrients in there!

PUREE FOODS. Even if you cook vegetables very well, they may still go down better if you puree them with a blender, such as an immersion blender. I'll talk more about kitchen gadgets on page 76. Again, you are trying to do the work outside of the stomach and break down foods as much as you can before you ingest them.

MAKE SMOOTHIES. Smoothies may be a way to still eat some fruits and vegetables uncooked, and since you've blended them into small particles, you may be better to able handle them.

LOW-FODMAP DIET

One popular diet that many GPers try is a low-FODMAP diet. FODMAP is an acronym from Fermentable, Oligo-, Di-, Mono-saccharides, and Polyols. These are all types of short-chain carbohydrates that, in some people, can be poorly absorbed. Crystal Saltrelli has seen the FODMAP diet work for many people. I have also talked with people where it didn't help, and I've talked with people who are able to eat some foods that are on this list. Again, you'll have to experiment.

In Appendix A, you'll find a chart of fruits and vegetables that are low and high FODMAP. Also, the recipes in this book indicate whether or not they are low FODMAP.

There are other categories of foods that can cause problems for people, such as histamines and glutamates. Histamines are often high in fermented foods, and glutamates are found in foods such as tomatoes, mushrooms, and gelatin.

Sometimes these categories can be really helpful, but I don't think it necessarily helps us to go into great detail about each of them in this book. There are a lot of great resources online, and I will include insights from some well-respected experts in the resources section.

2. FOOD TESTING

Now that we've discussed some possible problematic foods, the only way you will *really* know if something works or doesn't for you is to experiment. We are getting into food testing. Here is how you get started.

TRY MAKING BONE OR VEGGIE BROTH. This will be your foundation. After doing one or two days on broth and some known foods that work for you, continue with the following items on this list. Depending on how much you can ingest, you may have to really rest during this time. Take in what you can and be gentle with yourself.

KEEP A JOURNAL. Write down the times you eat food, how much you eat, and how you feel afterward for the next few hours to 24 hours.

THINK SIMPLE. Start with cooked, pureed food of one kind. Don't mix anything together in the beginning. Start with a small amount, depending on what you feel you can handle. For some, it might be a couple of bites; for others, it could be one-fourth cup.

CHEW, CHEW, CHEW! If you are eating solid foods, make sure you chew whatever you are eating extremely thoroughly. Chewing also means you have to take time to eat. Don't do anything else so you can concentrate and give your full attention to your food. Even if you are eating pureed food, chewing and swishing the food around your mouth is still a good idea, because you want to coat food particles with saliva. Your saliva has an enzyme in it called amylase that helps break down carbohydrates. If there are not obvious symptoms from eating something, the next day you can try eating another bite or another reasonable portion for your body.

EXPERIMENT WITH FOODS ONE AT A TIME. Try some healthy, fattier foods first, such as avocado, a tiny spoonful of coconut oil, pureed liver, or fish. These foods will provide you with more calories and nutrients, so if you can handle them, they will provide a good foundation to continue adding to.

DAILY JOURNAL WORKSHEET

Description: What did you eat?	Time Eaten	How much did you eat?	How did you feel afterward?

Once you have a good handle on what foods work for you, then you can start mixing and matching with care, and experimenting with different recipes.

The worksheet on page 69 will help guide you through a day in journaling and recording how things are making you feel so that you can make more informed decisions as you go along. You can also find blank copies of this worksheet at www.thenourishedbelly.com/downloads.

At the start of the day, access how you feel—on a scale of 1 to 10, 10 feeling great and 1 feeling at your worst, what would your number be? You can also use Spoon Theory (see page 5). If you think of each spoon as a unit of energy for a task, how many spoons do you have this morning? It might take a bit of experimenting to find a system that works for you.

At the end of the day, also ask yourself these questions:

- Based on your experiments today, what worked well for you?

- What would you change?

3. SUPPLEMENTATION

It's possible that you won't be able to eat enough in one day to get all of the nutrition that you need. I caution you to take supplements seriously. Anything you put into your body should be of high quality, and there should be a good reason why you are doing it. Many people just hear that something is good for them and they run out and purchase it, which can eventually be a waste of time and a waste of money. If you are working with a healthcare practitioner, it would be great to consult with them about which supplements would be best for you specifically, but below are a few general ones that I suggest.

AVAILABLE AT GROCERY STORES: New Chapter, MegaFood, NOW, Jarro, Carlsons, Nordic Naturals, and Garden of Life

AVAILABLE ONLINE OR THROUGH A PRACTITIONER: Standard Process, Thorne, Designs for Health, Innate Response, and Metagenics

Here are a few other supplements to think about using.

MULTIVITAMINS. Get a high-quality multivitamin from a reputable vitamin company. A liquid form might be a good option, depending on what you are able to digest.

VITAMIN B12. Remember from the discussion of stomach acid that it's necessary for your stomach to produce adequate stomach acid to absorb vitamin B12? A chemical called intrinsic factor is released by the parietal cells (where stomach acid comes from), and intrinsic factor binds to B12 and carries it down to the small intestine to be absorbed. It might be helpful to take a B12 supplement, especially if you test your levels with a healthcare practitioner and find you are B12 deficient. B12 is necessary for nerve health and brain health. Find a B12 supplement that dissolves under the tongue for better absorption. Also, you can go to a naturopathic doctor and get a B12 shot.

PROBIOTIC. One of the keys to overall health is to eat in a way that supports our beneficial gut bacteria. More and more information is coming out about the benefits of our gut bacteria. Many of them are involved in making some of our vitamins, supporting our immune system, and absorbing nutrients. One of the ways that we can support our gut bacteria, along with eating fermented foods when we can, is to take a probiotic. Probiotics support our digestion further down the gastrointestinal tract.

IBEROGAST. This German formula is created from a mix of different herbs that has been shown to reduce digestive symptoms. Iberogast has been used with some success in IBS and functional dyspepsia patients with increasing motility and improving gastrointestinal symptoms.[41]

Things to think about when choosing supplements:

- There are forms of supplements that are more absorbable than others. For example, iron citrate is a more absorbable form of iron than sulfate or fumarate.

- In general, you want to look for food-based supplements instead of synthetic vitamins. You can Google "the most absorbable form of ____."

- Look for vitamins that have been sourced from foods rather than made in the lab.

- Look for capsules or liquid forms of supplements; tablets are often harder to break down.

- Check with your healthcare provider if you have health issues; even supplements can interfere with your course of treatment.

PROTEIN POWDERS: Sometimes when making smoothies, it's helpful to add in a bit of protein powder to get some extra nutrients. Here's a list of protein powders suggested by fellow nutrition colleagues.

- Collagen hydrolysate from Great Lakes: I also talk about collagen hydrolysate when it comes to stocking the pantry, but it deserves a mention here in the protein powder category. I tend to favor this more than other protein powders because of the simplicity of ingredients. This is simply gelatin that has been processed to be easier to dissolve into liquids, hot and cold.

- Pea protein from Designs for Health: Designs for Health is a supplement company that only nutrition professionals have access to, or you can buy directly from their website.

41 B. Ottillinger, et al., "STW 5 (Iberogast)—A Safe and Effective Standard in the Treatment of Functional Gastrointestinal Disorders," *Wiener Medizinische Wochenschrift* (February 2013), DOI: 10.1007/s10354-012-0169-x.

According to my colleague, Michelle Dwyer, this protein powder is super smooth and doesn't have any weird taste.

- NutriBiotic Rice Protein: This is made from organic brown rice and also comes in a variety of flavors.

- Orgain: This company uses mostly organic ingredients, and I have tried the creamy chocolate fudge and vanilla flavors. I like the ingredients they use for the most part, but this powder does tend be on the sweeter side.

- HealthForce: HealthForce makes a variety of powders; you can mix and match different green powders, proteins, and nutrition blends. I like this company because they have a commitment to clean, green, and sustainable practices, and their powders come from whole food sources.

- Vega: Vega protein powders have a pretty clean ingredient list, but they can be pretty strong on the stevia front (to some people, stevia can be sickly sweet). The chocolate and the natural flavors are the least stevia saturated.

Personal Insight
Jennifer, 34, Berkeley

Jennifer first was diagnosed with eosinophilic esophagitis, and later, gastroparesis. I did an afternoon cooking lesson for her caregivers, showing them how to make bone broth, congee, and carrot ginger soup. Here is an update she gave me a month later.

"Hi Tammy. I have made progress!

I was having trouble with a distended belly, and last week my GI had me stop the eggs and almond milk, so I'm back on top 8 elimination[42]. Since I stopped, the belly bloating has decreased significantly.

---

42 A top 8 diet eliminates the top 8 most common allergens: dairy, eggs, wheat, tree nuts, peanuts, soy, fish, and shellfish.

However, my energy and my belly are improving, as long as I have a pureed soup (very basic) with the bone broth, some shredded chicken, rice, and zucchini. As long as I do this every day, my energy and mental clarity improve. Adding the rice really helps a lot; if it's just pureed veggies, it's difficult for me to digest. I've tried both ways (trial and error), and definitely the rice helps a lot!

It's been an interesting realization for me. I especially think my belly is trying to figure out what to do with solid foods after an all-liquid, processed foods diet. Which, honestly, were much easier on my gut, but they caused an unhealthy weight gain. All that processed starchy stuff packed on the pounds, but I never felt good; it was just what I could tolerate.

There was *lot* of discomfort going from an elemental liquid diet to solid foods. But the elemental formulas were not nutritious enough for me. I've quickly learned it's not about how many calories, it's the nutrients that make the difference. I do think the nutrient-dense soups are key for me and have been the biggest stepping stone to help me get here.

I can see now why my doctors have encouraged eating, not hustling on the G-Tube![43] Just like anything, your GI tract needs to be used. So transitioning from liquids to solids was very difficult. Now, my stomach is allowing more food. And I'm able to tolerate other foods much better! For example, breakfast is the meal I have the most ease with. I soak oats in coconut yogurt, milk, cinnamon, a tiny bit of coconut sugar, and vanilla. It's about two servings worth, and I have it with banana and a piece of turkey bacon.

Lunch has been my biggest struggle, with the most pain and difficulty. I was using a top 8 English muffin or a top 8 free roll, and I have a piece of turkey bacon, some turkey breast, and the soy-free, vegan cheese (just a little, for flavor).

---

43 A G-tube, which stands for gastrostomy tube, is a feeding tube that goes directly into the abdomen to deliver nutrition.

I had to cut the size in half to about 2.5 ounces, and it's helping a lot.

For dinner, I always have the 6 ounces of pureed broth soup.

Anyway, I wanted to let you know my progress!

It's a roller coaster, and I hope it continues to improve, but I take each moment that I feel better as a divine opportunity to feel good and *live!*

Thank you, so much!"

Chapter 5
PANTRY AND KITCHEN

In order to be ready to nourish yourself in your kitchen, think about getting some staples for your kitchen and pantry to make things much easier and more efficient. With pantry staples (which of course you have to test out) available, you can have things on hand that can help add nutrient density and flavor.

KITCHEN

SHARP KITCHEN KNIVES. There is nothing more frustrating than trying to cut with dull knives. They are serious time-wasters. If you have dull knives in your kitchen, it's worth getting them sharpened at your local hardware store. You can't just sharpen knives at home using the honer, which is that wand-looking thing that comes with your Thanksgiving carving set. Honers only keep sharp knives sharp. Don't forget to tuck in your fingers when you slice and chop things. It's worthwhile to watch a few videos on knife skills if you don't feel super comfortable in the kitchen. Just Google "knife skills" and some resources will pop up. Cutting things takes practice, so don't expect to feel good about it until you've had some time!

LARGE CUTTING BOARD. Bamboo is the new, more sustainable material used to make cutting boards. If you are able to eat garlic and onion, you might want to have a separate cutting board, as those flavors tend to linger, and garlic-flavored watermelon is not my favorite thing. Some people also like to have a separate cutting board for meats to prevent contamination when eating foods that you don't have to cook. Even though you are washing your cutting boards in hot soapy water, I like this idea and do it in my own kitchen.

SLOW COOKER. This is a must for you. In terms of convenience and work, a slow cooker is a huge lifesaver that cooks things slowly and at a low temperature. You almost can't mess up since you are cooking over a long period of time, which lets flavors gently melt into your meal. I use my slow cooker to make bone broth, braise meats, cook beans, and make soups. It's invaluable. There is a debate on the Internet about lead leaching in slow cooker glazes. There are people out there that look for slow cookers that are made of clay, glass, or stainless steel instead. I personally use a slow cooker that is not made out of these things, and have looked at the research and decided that at this point in my life and health, this is not something I'm going to concern myself with. You, who may have a compromised immune system and may not be absorbing all the nutrition you need, may want to look into getting alternative materials for your slow cooker.

BLENDER. A blender is also indispensable in the kitchen. While you are figuring out what works well for your body, blending up foods is extremely helpful. Be mindful that blending hot foods in a normal blender will cause pressure to build and the contents to explode outward—leave the spout open on top and pulse until smooth. Some people go big and get a Vitamix, which is one of the more powerful blenders out there. They also have a program for individuals that are going through medical hardship; if you apply, you can possibly get one donated to you. As of this writing, that program is temporarily suspended as they a have high demand, but it's worth checking out. Just Google "Vitamix donation" and you will find the page.

HAND BLENDER (IMMERSION BLENDER). This is also a must-have. I almost exclusively use a hand blender instead of a food processor because I like the easy cleanup. I use my hand blender to make dips, sauces, and creams like the Avocado Key Lime Pudding recipe on page 133. You can use it to make whipped cream as well. You'll also find it helpful for making the soups, like the Carrot Ginger Soup on page 102.

SPATULA. When you make a lot of sauces and dips, you want a spatula to scrape all that goodness out and not let anything go to waste!

SIEVE. A sieve is helpful for draining veggies after boiling or rinsing, and for making large batches of tea. Get a stainless steel one.

FUNNELS. As you start making more food in the kitchen, you'll want to start storing food either in the fridge or the freezer. Funnels can really help lessen cleanup and make sure more food or liquid makes it into your jars. In my kitchen, I have a stainless steel one that can fit into thin bottles for drinking teas, and then a larger one that fits into the mouth of my mason jars so that I can freeze and store my big pots of stews and soups without making a big mess.

MASON JARS. Mason jars have changed my kitchen. They are an excellent option for steering clear of plastic, especially when storing and heating food. If you still have plastic containers for storing food, recycle them! Instead, use multipurpose mason jars like Ball jars, which are made in the United States. You can drink directly out of them, freeze stuff in them (leave at least in inch on the top if you are freezing them), and use them to transport food. They are spill proof if you screw the lids on tightly, and they save space in the fridge. They also make great decorations, come in different sizes, and are great for storing dry pantry foods.

ELECTRIC KETTLE. If you are able to drink warm liquids and teas, an electric kettle makes things a lot easier. Electric kettles are a huge time-saver, and they'll turn themselves off when they are ready so you don't have to worry about getting up to turn off the kettle.

WATER FILTER. Having clean water is very important. We have a lot of stuff in our tap water that doesn't belong in our bodies. Chlorine and fluoride can be very damaging. I like the Multipure and Berkey water systems. Another investment, this will cost you between $300 to $400, but considering the amount of water you should be drinking, it's worth it. I also use filtered water when I'm making teas, soups, and stews.

PANTRY

There are a few basics when it comes to setting up your pantry that will help you make the recipes in this book and start transforming your pantry into a nutrition powerhouse. This includes both suggestions for your dry pantry and some ingredients that will keep in the fridge.

FRESH INGREDIENTS

MISO. Miso is one form of fermented soybean that holistic nutritionists often recommend. Unfermented soy can be difficult for some people to digest, and the fermentation process helps to neutralize some components that inhibit nutrient absorption. It's full of flavor and nutrients. Also, in its unheated form, it can be a nice dose of beneficial bacteria. I usually suggest mixing it in after a soup is removed from heat. Be sure to buy organic, since most conventional soy is genetically modified. Also, buy miso paste, which you'll find in the refrigerated section of grocery stores, not the powder. You can buy many different varieties, white miso is probably one of the mildest forms, and as a paste it can be stored in the fridge for quite a while, as long as it's stored in an airtight container and every time you scoop some out you use a clean spoon.

ORGANIC FRUITS AND VEGETABLES. Buy fruits and vegetables in small quantities. Think about what you are going to use in the next week. Often when things are about to go bad, you can throw them in the freezer, and when you are ready to make a nice veggie stock, you can bring your bag of veggies out. You can also buy frozen veggies and fruits; freezing is one of the best ways to preserve nutrients.

ALTERNATIVE MILKS. If you can handle milk, organic milk can be a possible source of good fats and protein. It's possible you might want to play around with the fat content. You can also buy nut milks; there are many different kinds that may work for you. Some possibilities are hemp milk, almond milk, and flax milk. Soy milk is not always recommended since it is unfermented and contains certain components that are hard to digest. However, you can say that with anything, so if you try soy milk and it works for you, then great. These milks are great to add to smoothies or drink on their own. Always look at the labels—they should have the least amount of ingredients.

ALMOND MEAL. Almond meal is an alternative flour that you can use to make a once-in-a-while treat, whether it be pancakes or muffins. Almond meal is from whole almonds. You will also see almond flour, which is made from blanched almonds with no skins. You can use either, although I may start with almond flour first, because without skins it will be lower fiber. Large servings of almond flour can be high FODMAP, so always start with smaller serving sizes and see how you respond. Almond, especially ground into meal, can go rancid easily, so store in a cool, dark place or in the fridge.

SHELF-STABLE INGREDIENTS

COCONUT OIL. I use coconut oil often in my kitchen to sauté veggies, to use in baking, and to moisturize my skin when need be. If you can handle coconut oil, it's a lovely way to add fat and calories; plus, coconut oil has other nutrients that are helpful to the body. According to Rebecca Wood, author of *The New Whole Foods Encyclopedia*, coconut oil is one of the few plant sources of lauric acid, which is also in breast milk and enhances brain and immune system function.[44] It's also proven to be antiviral, antibacterial, and antifungal.

AVOCADO OIL. Avocado oil is another monounsaturated fat that has a milder flavor. Some people prefer to cook with avocado oil instead of coconut oil for this reason.

EXTRA-VIRGIN OLIVE OIL. Olive oil is a monounsaturated fat and is great for adding flavor. I often drizzle it on soups and veggies, and sometimes use it for cooking when I know I'm not frying anything. Heating olive oil too high can damage the oil and thus be damaging for your health. Extra-virgin olive oil is the first pressing of the olives, so is the best tasting and provides the most nutrients. I would stick to buying extra virgin and drizzle after cooking to maintain flavor.

GHEE. Ghee is a traditional fat that comes to us by way of India. Ghee is clarified butter, which means all the protein solids have been taken out, and it is pure fat. It's expensive to buy at the store but super simple to make at home. (You'll find the recipe on page 94.) I think it smells like a fresh buttered croissant, and it gives your dishes this aroma! Pretty much anything cooked in ghee is heavenly. If you are going to fry anything, ghee is a great choice since it has an extremely high melting point.

Nutrient-Dense Additions

KELP POWDER. Kelp is another name for seaweed, but you'll find kelp powder in the supplement section of a natural foods store. It's high in minerals and is great sprinkled on to savory dishes.

COCOA POWDER. Cocoa powder is powdered chocolate liquor that contains 10 to 22 percent cocoa butter.[45] It is full of flavonoids, a type of antioxidant that is helpful for healing and repair in the body. I use it to make baked goods, chocolate puddings, and hot chocolate. For some people, cocoa powder can be stimulating, so if you are sensitive to caffeine at all, be mindful of your intake. Also, it is high

---

44 Rebecca Wood, *The New Whole Foods Encyclopedia*, (New York: Penguin Books, 2010).
45 Michael Murray, *The Encyclopedia of Healing Foods*, (New York: Atria Books, 2005).

in arginine, which is an amino acid that can exacerbate any active herpes infections. Store in an airtight container in a cool, dark place.

ALGAE. Algae are single-celled, photosynthetic organisms that grow in freshwater lakes and ponds. Two specific types of algae, spirulina and chlorella, contain bioavailable essential fatty acids, chlorophyll, active enzymes, vitamins, minerals, complex sugars, and phytonutrients, and help with heavy-metal detox.

SPIRULINA (BLUE-GREEN ALGAE). Spirulina grows naturally in lakes that have a high acidity. It is free-forming and floats on the surface of the water. One of the most primitive forms of plant life, spirulina was used by the Aztecs and some Africans as an important food staple. Spirulina is up to 77 percent a complete and readily digestible protein. It is cooling and detoxifying, and supports all organ functions. It lowers cholesterol, enhances the immune system, and is also cancer protective. It helps digestion by increasing beneficial bacteria.

CHLORELLA. Chlorella was the first plant to grow with a true nucleus and has been on earth for more than 2.5 billion years. Chlorella is a superior source of assimilable chlorophyll, which helps to cleanse and detoxify cells in the body. A clean and healthy cell can better utilize other nutrients. It is helpful for chronic gastritis, high blood pressure, diabetes, constipation, anemia, and high cholesterol. Chlorella is similar to spirulina, but has less protein and more chlorophyll. It contains all essential amino and fatty acids and is very rich in lysine. One teaspoon has 6 grams of protein.

SEAWEED. Sea vegetables are one of the most nutritious foods you could eat. Most famous in Asian cultures, they are also used by people from Irish cultures, the Inuit, and other coastal peoples. They are incredibly mineral rich, with the mineral content being 7 to 38 percent of their dry weight.

They help to reduce blood cholesterol, remove radioactive and metallic elements from the body, support the thyroid, counter obesity, strengthen bones, teeth, and nerve function, and help improve digestion. The most significant elements are calcium, iodine, phosphorus, sodium, and iron. Seaweed is a rich protein source, containing up to 38 percent protein. It is also an above average source of vitamins A and B.

The easiest way to use seaweed is to cook it in broths and soups. A popular type to buy is called kombu or wakame, and when simmered in your soup or broth, you are getting some great nutrition in your food. You can experiment with different kinds.

GELATIN. I'll talk more about gelatin when I discuss bone broth on page 87. What's exciting about gelatin is that you can buy it in powdered form. Gelatin is what you can use to make gelatin desserts, and also what you can add to soups and stews to make them more nutrient dense. There are two types you can buy: gelatin and collagen hydrolysate. Collagen hydrolysate dissolves more easily in liquids and is nice when stirred into smoothies. It will never firm up when cooled. Gelatin, however, must be dissolved in warm water and will gel in cooler temperatures. They are both a good source of protein and can be easier to digest. I prefer the brands Great Lakes Gelatin and Vital Proteins. Start with a small dose and work your way up if there is no stomach upset.

TAPIOCA FLOUR. I wouldn't necessarily consider tapioca flour the most nutrient dense of flours, but it's low FODMAP, an alternative to wheat flour, and it can help make some fun snacks. Tapioca flour comes from the cassava root, which pops up in many, many cultures around the world. It has a somewhat chewy consistency when baked. You may be familiar with tapioca in the form of the small, chewy balls in Asian bubble tea. But you will also see cassava as yucca in South America, and it is generally one of the main carbohydrate sources in tropical regions. For your purposes, tapioca flour will be included in a recipe for a Brazilian cheese bread called Pão de Queijo (page 129). Wear an apron when you use it—it can get all over the place!

Herbs that Aid Digestion

Herbs are another important addition to your pantry. Some herbs can help to enhance motility and can provide some relief for nausea and bloating. Again, you must test these foods and herbs to make sure they agree with your body. Below are just a few, but there are many more herbs that can help with digestion. You can take them in supplement form, put them into broths, or buy them dry to steep as teas. You can find many resources online (search for "herbs for digestion") and also find many books that focus on Western and Eastern herbalism. Consult with a medical practitioner before adding any supplements or herbs to your diet.

CARMINATIVES. Carminatives are herbs that can help to relieve gas and bloating. They have volatile oils in them that can increase gastric emptying and can encourage peristalsis throughout the digestive tract, therefore releasing gas.

ANISE. Anise is the flavor that lends sweetness to black licorice. It is a digestive aid. It acts as a carminative and can be used as leaves to simmer in a pot, or its seeds can be ground into desserts. *Caution:* Not recommended during pregnancy.

CARDAMOM. Cardamom has a sweet smell and goes well when mixed with ginger and cinnamon. You can simmer entire pods in dishes and remove them right before serving.

GINGER. Ginger is a root that is native to India and likes to grow in hot, tropical weather. I've heard from many GPers that ginger chews help during flare-ups. Ginger helps with nausea, is anti-inflammatory, and is supportive to the immune system. It can also reduce gas and bloating. Look for fresh ginger; simply cutting a few slices and steeping them in hot water can create a delicious tea. *Caution:* Ginger does have blood-thinning actions, so be mindful if on blood thinners. Please consult your doctor.

PEPPERMINT. Peppermint is a muscle relaxant and can help to dispel gas and relieve an upset stomach. *Caution:* Peppermint is not recommended for those suffering from acid reflux, as it can relax the sphincter that prevents food from coming back up into esophagus.

Chapter 6
RECIPES

The recipes in this book are based on the idea of simplicity. There are few ingredients, many of which can be substituted out if need be. The way to approach these recipes is to make them, or cut them in half to make a small amount, and then test it out. Take a bite and see how you feel. When you are ready, take another bite. Recipes are labeled for allergens. Some have options that will make them either dairy free or low FODMAP. Look for notes in the ingredient sections for optional ingredients. Most do not contain soy, except for recipes that use miso.

 Gluten Free

 Dairy Free

LOW FOD MAP   Low FODMAP

HEALING BASICS

BONE BROTH

Broth is an extremely mineral-rich food found in culinary traditions around the world, and if liquids work for you, then broth is an incredible addition to your rotation.

You'll find a bone broth–based soup or stew in pretty much any culture's culinary cuisine. It's often prescribed to build up strength, and it's at the foundation of the popular Gut and Psychology Syndrome (GAPS) diet for those who need to rebuild their gut lining. Let's take a look at why it's so powerful.

HIGH IN MINERALS. Due to the lack of minerals in soils on conventional farms and the current American state of health, most people are deficient in minerals. Minerals are just as important as vitamins to your daily bodily functions. Bones are a powerhouse of minerals. In *Nourishing Broth*, Kaayla Daniel and Sally Fallon Morell state that bones are made up of 50 percent mineral content.[46] Through prolonged simmering, you can extract all of these precious nutrients. Thomas Cowan, one of the authors of *The Fourfold Path to Healing*, suggests that adding bone broth to your diet is the fastest way to rebuild your mineral deposits.

AN IMPORTANT SOURCE OF GELATIN. Bone broth does not always come out gelatinous since it depends on the age of the animal and the way you make your broth. However, when your broth gels when cooled, you know you have liquid gold! Gelatin is the culinary word for collagen, and collagen is what makes up 25 to 35 percent of the body's total protein.[47] Collagen is responsible for holding your body together—literally. It acts as the glue that keeps your muscles, joints, and cell structures in place. You can think of the glue as losing its

---

46 Sally Fallon Morell and Kaayla T. Daniel, *Nourishing Broth: An Old-Fashioned Remedy for the Modern World*, (New York: Grand Central Lifestyle, 2014).
47 Ibid.

effectiveness as you age, and thus, you can break apart more easily. Not an awesome image, but makes sense, right?

The nutrients in bone broth are great for your joints. One of the primary ways your joints are protected is by the synovial fluid that surrounds your joint cavities. Through movement, synovial fluid moves in and out of the joint capsule while providing nutrients you need to maintain joint health and also cushioning your joints from impact.

Hydration and optimum nutrition are also important to this process. One way to maintain all the different components of synovial fluid is to drink plenty of broth. Broth, especially gelatinous broth, is full of the building blocks of synovial fluid. You've probably heard of the effectiveness of glucosamine and chondroitin sulfate when it comes to joint health. Broth provides natural sources of both these nutrients.

Gelatin is an important food on its own (see page 83); the Soothing Sweetened Jellies recipe on page 135 is a good way to get your dose of gelatin.

HEALING AND REGENERATIVE. Gelatinous broth is an excellent digestive aid and is extremely healing to your gut, nervous system, and entire body. This is the original reason that sweetened gelatin is served in hospitals. Patients were served a gelatin-based food, but in the words of *Full Moon Feast* author Jessica Prentice, the version served to patients nowadays is a "toxic mimic" of tradition.

Broth is not a complete protein, primarily missing tryptophan, but it has some important amino acids. Included in the large amino acid profile of bone broth are glycine, proline, and glutamine.

Glycine is necessary in creating glucose when you are in need of more energy and is vital in supporting your detoxification pathways (thus, cleansing with only bone broth is a great idea).

Proline is essential for the production of collagen, which helps maintain healthy skin, bones, ligaments, tendons, and cartilage.

Glutamine is important for gut health, as it helps to feed entero-cytes, which absorb digested food and transport nutrients to the bloodstream. Glutamine helps to keep the integrity of the gut lining, which is now seen as preventing food allergies and possibly being tied to mood disorders.

Bone broth can be used by itself as a snack, with a little miso, and is a fabulous base for soups and stews. I suggest my clients use it instead of water to cook rice or any grain. Adding just a splash to stir-fries not only supplies nutrients, but flavor.

BONE BROTH

Bone broth is super simple to make, trust me! Sometimes it takes people time to figure out where to buy bones (most local grocery stores and farmer's markets will have bones), and just the act of doing it the first time can be an obstacle. But once you do it, it's easy, and it's one of the staples that underlies a nutrient-dense diet. You can mix bones, but I usually keep my chicken bones separate since the flavors can be different.

Makes roughly 3 to 4 quarts

1 to 2 pounds bones

2 to 3 quarts filtered water

2 tablespoons apple cider vinegar

1 medium yellow onion, roughly chopped

4 carrots, including tops, roughly chopped

4 stalks celery, roughly chopped

2 bay leaves

1 Place the bones at the bottom of a stockpot or slow cooker. Cover the bones with filtered water.

2 Add the apple cider vinegar. The vinegar will help to pull the minerals from the bones.

3 Bring the broth to a boil and then reduce to a simmer.

4 Follow the cooking times below.

5 In the last 4 hours, add onion, carrots, celery, and bay leaves.

6 When finished, strain and funnel the broth into jars

7 Freeze some (label with the date and kind of broth), and keep some in the fridge for immediate use

- Fish (keep the fish heads!): minimum 20 minutes, no more than 1 hour
- Chicken: 12 to 24 hours (See Whole Chicken Broth, page 91.)
- Lamb and goat: 36 hours
- Pork and beef: 36 to 48 hours

WHOLE CHICKEN BROTH

Chicken broth is usually the broth that I tell people to start with, since getting chicken bones can be relatively easy. Many butchers have chicken backs, heads, and feet for sale at a relatively cheap price, and these are *great* bones for making broth. You can also buy chicken with the bone in, or save your bones if someone in your household roasts a chicken. Roasted bones take on an extra flavor.

Makes 4 quarts

1 whole chicken

4 quarts filtered water, divided

2 tablespoons apple cider vinegar

1 medium yellow onion, roughly chopped

4 medium carrots, including tops, roughly chopped

4 stalks celery, roughly chopped

2 bay leaves

1 Place whole chicken into stockpot or slow cooker.

2 Cover completely with the first 2 quarts of water and add the apple cider vinegar.

3 Simmer for 4 to 6 hours.

4 Take out the chicken then pull meat from the bones. Careful, it's hot!

5 Store the meat in the fridge for use throughout the week.

6 Place the bones back into the broth, and place another 2 quarts of water in.

7 Simmer for another 12 to 24 hours. In the last 4 hours, place in the onion, carrots, celery, and bay leaves.

8 Strain and store in glass jars.

VEGGIE MINERAL BROTH

GF DF LOW FOD MAP

Making a great veggie broth is simple, nutritious, and hydrating. It's full of minerals from yummy vegetables. At my nutrition school in Bauman College, we made a three-layer veggie broth. It started with root veggies (sweet potatoes, carrots, parsnips, potatoes), next had leafy greens (kale, collards, spinach), and ended with booster foods (mushrooms, seaweed). Booster foods are any foods that you can add to a meal that will boost the nutrition. I love to have a cup in the morning first thing when I wake up. I'll often keep it in a thermos that I can sip throughout the day. They are a fantastic source of minerals and an excellent way to use veggie scraps in your kitchen. Save your veggie scraps for this recipe—kale stems, pepper tops, asparagus ends, corn cobs, carrot tops. Keep everything in a bag in the freezer until you get about 3 to 4 loosely-packed cups.

Makes 2 to 3 quarts

BASIC INGREDIENTS

1 yellow onion, roughly chopped

2 to 3 medium to large carrots, roughly chopped

3 to 4 medium celery stalks, roughly chopped

2 to 3 quarts filtered water

OPTIONAL INGREDIENTS

3 to 4 cups veggie scraps, roughly chopped

1 to 2 sweet potatoes, roughly chopped

1 winter squash, roughly chopped

1 cup mushrooms (any kind), roughly chopped

handful whole seaweed

1 bunch kale, roughly chopped

1 Throw everything into a stockpot or slow cooker and cover with the filtered water.

2 Simmer for 3 to 4 hours

3 Strain, and store!

4 Freeze some in mason jars (don't fill the jars too full) and put some in the fridge for immediate use (in the next 4 or 5 days).

5 Use it for making grains and stir-fries, or just having a cup with a little salt as a snack.

SIMPLE MISO SOUP

Miso is a fermented soy product. If you are sensitive at all to soy, go ahead and skip this recipe. This can be a simple soup that if you are in a pinch, you can make with just some warm water and miso paste. Remember, miso can provide a nice dose of healthy probiotics, protein, and other nutrients. You can adjust the amount of miso you prefer; some people like a more miso-heavy taste in the broth. Also, you can make a more substantial soup with rice or pureed veggies. Add the miso in at the very end following the steps below.

Makes 1 serving

1 cup filtered water

1 teaspoon miso paste

1 Bring the cup of water to a boil in a small saucepan over medium heat. Turn off the heat.

2 Add the miso paste.

3 Mix until thoroughly combined.

4 Pour into a small bowl or mug to sip, and enjoy!

GARLIC-INFUSED GHEE

Some people who normally don't do well with dairy can eat ghee, since the lactose has been removed. Ghee is something simple to make, and you can add some herbs to get in a bit more nutrition.

Especially if you are on a low-FODMAP diet, garlic-infused ghee might be a way you can sneak that flavor back into some of your dishes. Of course, you can make this without garlic and have plain ghee as well. Using ghee in some of your recipes will also help make the nutrients in your food more absorbable.

I usually don't make large batches of ghee at once. I use it pretty frequently, so I keep it in my pantry, which keeps it soft and easy to scoop out. After 3 or 4 months, ghee loses its nutty aroma and starts to smell stale, so try to use it within 2 months. Relish using ghee: It has a long history and is extremely nourishing. It will add a beautiful flavor to your meals and a foundation of clean, wholesome nutrition to your diet.

Makes 2 cups

3 sticks unsalted organic butter

4 cloves garlic, roughly chopped (optional)

1 teaspoon thyme (optional)

1 teaspoon rosemary (optional)

1 teaspoon basil (optional)

1 In a saucepan, heat the butter, garlic (if using), and herbs (if using) on low until the mixture starts to simmer. A white foam will rise to the top, and it should start to bubble.

2 When the foam starts to subside, tilt the saucepan to check the color of the solids at the bottom. Roughly 15 minutes after the start of simmering, they should turn golden brown, and the ghee will be done. Be careful not to burn the solids on the bottom, as this will affect the flavor.

3 Strain and place in an opaque glass jar.

4 Store the ghee in a cool, dark place.

NOURISHING RICE PORRIDGE (CONGEE)

Congee is a complete comfort food for me. My family used to eat it on Sunday mornings with side dishes of dried pork, pickled vegetables, and fish. In reality, this is a dish that can be eaten at any time of day. Congee is often recommended for anyone who needs to rehabilitate and eat something easily digestible. You'll find a rice porridge in other cultures as well; in Korea it's called *jook*, and in my Taiwanese family, we call it *mwueh*.

Makes 6 to 8 servings

2 cups day-old rice (if you use uncooked rice, let it cook for longer)

1 quart bone broth or vegetable broth

2 strips kombu

2 cups water (if needed)

1 On the stovetop, combine the rice, broth, and seaweed in a large saucepan, and bring to a simmer. You can also use a slow cooker, place everything inside, and let sit overnight.

2 Stir every 10 minutes or so, adding water as needed to keep the congee from sticking to the bottom of the pot.

3 Cook until you are happy with the consistency, usually around an hour.

BOILED YUCCA

GF | LOW FOD MAP

Yucca is another name for cassava, which is a tuber that feeds much of the world. Other names are tapioca and manioc. Yucca is mainly carbohydrate, and it's high in manganese and vitamin C. It cannot be eaten raw. It's amazing how boiling will change this inedible tuber into something so nutritious. It's very, very simple to prepare. You can make this into a mash, or you can boil it until it's as soft as you like.

You can try boiling this in broth, as yucca will absorb the flavor of whatever liquid it's in. It's up to you if you want to add butter, ghee, or coconut oil at the end.

Makes 2 servings

2 to 3 cups filtered water or broth

1 medium yucca, peeled and sliced into half circle pieces roughly an inch thick

salt, to taste

1 teaspoon butter, ghee, or coconut oil (use coconut oil for a DF option)

1 In a medium saucepan or pot, heat the water/broth on medium heat.

2 Place the yucca into the liquid and bring to a simmer. Cover and simmer for 30 to 40 minutes. A fork should slide easily through each piece.

3 Strain and salt to taste. Add butter, ghee, or coconut oil if desired.

CREAMY POLENTA

`GF`

Made from corn, polenta is normally made in a 1 to 4 ratio of grain to liquid. Here we are using 5 cups of liquid (you can use 5 cups of broth, or even water if you decide to forgo adding milk) because you want this to lean more toward the consistency of porridge, which also spreads out the fiber content. Polenta cooks extremely quickly, so for days when you might not be feeling great, it won't be a lot of trouble to ask someone to make this for you. Stir it from time to time so that it won't stick on the bottom. You can also use broth to make it more tasty and nutrient dense.

Polenta goes well with many foods. You can scramble an egg on top or eat it with a bit of avocado to add a bit of healthy fat. Just be mindful to eat it in small amounts to make sure that your stomach agrees.

Makes 5 cups

3½ cups veggie or bone broth

1½ cups cow's milk, light coconut milk, or alternative milk (optional)

1 teaspoon salt

1 cup polenta

1 Bring liquid, milk (if using), and salt to a boil in a medium saucepan. Slowly stir in polenta.

2 Simmer for roughly 15 minutes and stir frequently to keep polenta from sticking to the bottom.

3 Remove from heat and serve or store. You can spread the polenta onto a cookie sheet and wait until it is cooled to cut into squares, and either freeze or put in the fridge.

4 Reheat by simply frying the cuts, or add more liquid until you have the consistency you want.

NOURISHING MEALS

When eating smoothies or soups, be sure to mix a bit in your mouth so that parts of your food are mixed in with saliva. Saliva contains enzymes that are important for digesting carbohydrates.

Also, you can add the following ingredients to smoothies and soups for extra nutrients and protein, if you test them out separately.

- 1 tablespoon collagen hydrolysate. To test, mix 1 teaspoon in ½ cup of water and drink.

- ½ teaspoon coconut oil or flax oil. To test, try with ¼ teaspoon and take directly. If this seems too much, try less.

- You can also think about adding ginger to any of them, either in slices that you take out before eating or blended into your puree.

POWER SMOOTHIE

Smoothies are a way to blend food, breaking down fruits and vegetables to make them a little more digestible. It's also a way to add a few more nutrients in a pureed form. You can make this dairy free by taking out the yogurt, and low FODMAP by not having peaches or pears.

Serves 2

1 banana

1 cup seasonal fruit, such as berries, peaches, or pears (skins off)

½ cup light coconut milk or ½ cup plain whole yogurt

1 handful spinach or other leafy green

1 tablespoon protein powder

dash kelp powder

dash spirulina or chlorella

filtered water

Place all ingredients into a blender and blend. Add water until you get the desired consistency.

SWEET MILLET CEREAL

Millet is a nutty-tasting grain that is a wonderful addition to the breakfast porridge rotation. It's one of the grains with a higher protein content compared to corn and rice, and is also a good source of minerals and B vitamins.

Those with hypothyroid shouldn't consume millet on a regular basis, since it has a substance that can interfere with thyroid function.

Makes 3 cups

½ cup millet

2 cups filtered water

1 cup coconut milk or alternative milk

1 banana, sliced

1 egg

1 tablespoon chia seeds (optional)

2 teaspoons maple syrup

¹⁄₁₆ teaspoon sea salt

1 Place the millet in a medium saucepan with the water and coconut milk.

2 Add in the banana. Simmer with a lid on for 20 to 25 minutes.

3 Stir in the egg, chia seeds (if using), maple syrup, and salt.

4 Let sit, covered, for 5 to 10 minutes.

5 Experiment with different toppings, and enjoy!

ALMOND FLOUR BANANA SQUASH PANCAKES

These almond flour pancakes are a nice alternative to wheat flour pancakes, and they are good hot or cold. They are denser than normal pancakes, so don't expect the same fluffiness, but they are wonderful in their own way. My favorite way to eat them is to dip them in yogurt with a touch of maple syrup.

The vanilla and cinnamon are optional. If you aren't ready to add them to the recipe, try the recipe without them first and see how your stomach reacts. Also, if you are using canned pumpkin, add a touch more almond meal. Canned pumpkin can be a little wetter than home-cooked squash. I prefer to use roasted kabocha squash in this recipe.

Makes 6 small pancakes

1 ripe banana

2 eggs

⅛ teaspoon vanilla extract (optional)

2 heaping tablespoons cooked squash or canned pumpkin

½ cup almond meal

⅛ teaspoon ground cinnamon (optional)

⅛ teaspoon salt

⅛ teaspoon baking powder

3 tablespoons coconut oil or butter

jam, maple syrup, or yogurt, to top

1 Mash the banana, eggs, vanilla (if using), and squash in a medium bowl with an immersion blender or mixer.

2 Heat a large sauté pan on the stove while you add the almond meal, cinnamon (if using), salt, and baking powder. Mix thoroughly with a spatula.

3 Turn heat to low and place 1 tablespoon of coconut oil or butter per batch in the sauté pan.

4 Cook for roughly 5 minutes on each side. Look for firmness on the bottom before you flip. Be careful flipping!

5 Enjoy with jam or maple syrup.

CARROT GINGER SOUP

Carrot ginger soup is a classic soup, and so beautiful and colorful that it's a joy to eat. Simmering this soup with chunks of ginger helps to flavor the dish with a lovely ginger flavor that is cited by many GPers to help with nausea and settling the tummy. Making this with a bone broth or veggie broth will add both flavor and nutrients. I like to add a bit of coconut milk, which no longer makes it low FODMAP, but the bit of fat will help to absorb nutrients, so test it out. You could also add a teaspoon of flax oil or coconut oil, which are FODMAP friendly.

Makes 4 servings

2 large carrots, roughly chopped

1 quart broth or filtered water

1 small claw ginger, sliced into large pieces

1½ teaspoons coconut milk or flax seed oil (optional)

salt, to taste

1 In a medium saucepan, place in one quart broth or filtered water, and add in chopped carrots and ginger.

2 Over medium heat, bring to a simmer.

3 Cover with a lid and simmer for 20 minutes, or until carrots are soft.

4 Remove pieces of ginger.

5 Using an immersion blender, blend carrots until soup is smooth.

6 Add coconut milk or flax seed oil, if desired.

7 Add salt to taste.

8 Enjoy!

SUMMER SQUASH SOUP

In this soup, use any type of summer squash, such as zucchini, yellow summer squash, crooknecks, or patty pans. Packed with nutrients, these yummy veggies supply antioxidants that include loads of carotenes. When purchasing, look for skin that is smooth and without punctures. Try peeling the squash to lower fiber content—see if it affects digestion. It's possible you will be OK with the skins, as they are on the softer side.

Makes 4 servings

1 quart broth or filtered water

1 teaspoon coconut oil or ghee

2 to 3 medium summer squashes, deseeded and cut lengthwise

1 medium tomato, cut into large chunks (optional)

½ cup cooked rice (optional)

1 tablespoon collagen hydrolysate (optional)

sea salt and pepper, to taste

1 tablespoon olive oil

1 teaspoon lemon juice

1 Pour broth or water in a large saucepan over medium heat. Turn off when a simmer begins.

2 Place a medium sauté pan over medium heat. When warm, put in the coconut oil or ghee and allow it to melt.

3 Throw the summer squashes and tomato (if using) into the sauté pan. Sauté for roughly 3 to 4 minutes. You may add in a bit of broth or water and cover to allow it to cook faster. The pieces should turn more opaque and be easily forked.

4 When cooked, add the summer squashes and tomato into the broth. Add the rice here as well, if using.

5 Using an immersion blender, blend until smooth.

6 Add collage hydrolysate, if using.

7 Add the salt and pepper.

8 Pour into bowls and drizzle with olive oil and a squeeze of lemon. Serve immediately, or, when preparing for future use, add olive oil and lemon juice when serving.

KABOCHA MISO SOUP

This is one of my favorite soups. Winter squash by itself is such a treat, and blended with broth plus a little coconut milk (if it agrees with you) is fantastic. There's something about the coconut-and-squash combo that is so satisfying. This recipe uses uncooked squash, but if you have squash leftover, this soup is even quicker to make. You can use any squash, but kabocha is one of my favorites. You can even mix the different kinds together! For added flavor, add 1 medium yellow onion (high-FODMAP). Feel free to replace the coconut oil with butter.

Makes 3 to 4 servings

1 medium green, orange, or gray kabocha squash, deseeded and halved

1 tablespoon coconut oil

½ teaspoon minced ginger, or 1 small claw of ginger, cut into large pieces

1 quart chicken broth

1 tablespoon collagen hydrolysate (optional)

2 tablespoons miso paste

¼ to ½ teaspoon sea salt

1 Preheat the oven to 400°F.

2 Line a baking sheet with parchment paper on top and place kabocha facedown.

3 Bake for 30 minutes or until you can easily put a fork through the squash.

4 Remove from oven and scoop the inside of the squash out, discarding the skin. (Normally, the skin is edible.)

5 Heat a sauté pan on medium.

6 Place the coconut oil in the pan. Add the ginger. Sauté for 4 to 5 minutes or until the onion is translucent.

7 In a large saucepan, pour in the broth, onion, ginger, miso, hydrolysate if using, and kabocha.

8 Using an immersion blender, blend until smooth in the saucepan.

9 Bring contents to a simmer. Add filtered water if you would like a thinner consistency.

10 Add salt, to taste, and serve.

SUMMERTIME GAZPACHO

Gazpacho originates from the southern region of Spain, as I first learned in high school Spanish class when my first thought was, "cold soup?" However, the first time someone made it for me from fresh ingredients, I was forever changed. It's a perfect hot, sunny day dish, and when you make it with ingredients available at the peak of the summer season, you can't go wrong.

The three main vegetables are low in fiber individually, but together they will provide a bit more. Again, you can halve this recipe or share with someone and start with a small serving to see how you handle it. This is one of the few raw recipes that I include because it really is so delicious, and everything is blended. You could also heat this soup up to see if it goes down a bit easier. If you decide to heat it up, you could put in a few whole garlic cloves and take them out before eating to add a bit of garlic flavor.

Makes 3 to 4 servings

1½ pounds (roughly 5 medium) ripe tomatoes, chopped

1 medium yellow or red bell pepper, roughly chopped

1 medium cucumber, peeled and roughly chopped

1 teaspoon balsamic vinegar

¾ teaspoon salt

2 tablespoons extra-virgin olive oil, plus more to garnish (optional)

black pepper, to taste

avocado, to garnish (optional)

1 Combine all of the ingredients in a food processor or blender and pulse until finely chopped.

2 Pour into a bowl.

3 Cover and chill for a few hours before serving. Garnish with the avocado and olive oil, or as desired.

CORN SOUP

GF DF LOW FOD MAP

Eating straight corn is not GP friendly, as it is actually quite high in fiber. However, that doesn't mean that you can't enjoy the sweetness and deliciousness of corn. You could also substitute other high-fiber vegetables that you enjoy but can't eat. For example, you could simmer broccoli here instead of corn, just to get the flavor, and remove it before eating.

This is actually a version of a Taiwanese corn soup, without the corn kernels. I don't advise using veggie broth as a base, only because it takes away from the corn flavor. I love using a bone broth, which adds dimension and all those important nutrients as well. The eggs add a little protein, body, and creaminess, and depending on how you stir, they will make a creamy broth or should wisp like egg drop soup. Start with just a splash of coconut milk, and if it works for you, increase the amount slowly. Enjoy!

Makes 1 quart

1 quart bone broth or filtered water

2 whole cobs corn, broken as necessary to fit into pot

2 whole eggs

½ cup light coconut milk, optional (I like the Native Forest brand)

⅛ tablespoon sea salt

1 Place the broth or filtered water into a slow cooker or large saucepan on the stove over medium heat.

2 Add in corn cobs.

3 Bring to a simmer when it starts to boil. Allow to simmer for 20 minutes.

4 Add coconut milk, if desired.

5 Crack eggs into a bowl and stir until combined.

6 Take out corn cobs and compost.

7 Turn off heat and pour in egg mixture while using a fork or whisk to rapidly whisk it in. (For more eggy tendrils, like egg drop soup, whisk in slowly.)

8 Add salt, adjusting to taste.

9 Enjoy some and store some for later.

VERMICELLI NOODLE SOUP `GF` `DF` `LOW FOD MAP`

I grew up eating noodles. They are quick and satisfying, and vermicelli (bean thread) noodles, while not the most nutrient-dense option, help to shake things up. When paired with bone broth, the noodles can still be part of a nutritious diet. I keep vermicelli noodles in my pantry when I need something quick and find my pantry to be a little bare. You'll need two saucepans, one to boil the noodles, the other to heat up the broth and boil the greens.

Makes 1 serving

1 quart chicken broth

2 cups filtered water

1 package vermicelli noodles

1 cup roughly cut spinach or bok choy

1 egg

1 Fill one medium saucepan halfway with filtered water and set to boil.

2 Fill a second medium saucepan with the broth and also set to boil.

3 When the water starts to boil, add the vermicelli noodles; they should be a bit bigger than the size of your fist. (Or, you could always cook more and keep them in the fridge for more noodle soup.) Boil for 2 to 3 minutes.

4 Taste for doneness. They should break apart easily, but not be mushy. Drain the noodles and set aside.

5 When the broth starts to boil, add the greens and simmer for 1 to 2 minutes.

6 Crack open the egg and add it to the broth. You can stir the egg in or simply cover and turn off the heat.

7 Serve in bowls, add the desired amount of noodles, and enjoy!

DAIKON SOUP

This dish is inspired by my mother's home cooking and my eating lots and lots of daikon radish growing up. Daikon is delightfully light and comforting at the same time, especially when it's cooked in soups. It's also considered to be detoxifying, anti-inflammatory, and full of nutrients. It's extremely soft when cooked thoroughly and retains a sweet, light flavor. The recipe below is simply a guide, but include whatever you want and add more miso if you want it saltier!

Makes 4 servings

1 medium daikon radish, chopped in 1-inch cubes

1 handful dried wakame

1 quart chicken broth

1 tablespoon miso paste, plus more to taste (optional)

sea salt, to taste

1 Place daikon radish and wakame into a medium stockpot with 2 quarts of broth.

2 Simmer for roughly 30 to 40 minutes, until daikon cubes are translucent and a fork goes easily through them.

3 If using miso, follow directions below. If not, then salt to taste.

4 In a small cup, ladle out one-half cup of the heated broth, and add the miso paste. Stir until dissolved and add into soup.

5 Dissolve another teaspoon the same way until the desired saltiness and taste is acquired.

6 Enjoy!

BASIC AREPAS

I traveled to Colombia when I was younger and one of the foods that I really enjoyed were arepas. Made from corn, they are filled with delicious ingredients, and you can place any matter of toppings on top.

For your case, arepas can be a source of calories and nutrients, and something that can easily be made bite size. In this recipe, broth adds more nutrients, but you can also make this with water, or, if you can handle it, cow's milk or coconut milk.

If you are very sensitive to fats, you can place a bit of water or broth in a pan and steam these.

Makes 8 servings

1 cup masa harina

1 cup filtered water, broth, or any type of milk

1 teaspoon salt

1 tablespoon ghee (use coconut oil for DF option)

1 Place the masa harina, liquid, and salt in a large mixing bowl. Mix with your hands until combined.

2 Allow to sit for 10 minutes. The dough should solidify to make it easier to handle, but it will look roughly like the consistency of pancake batter.

3 Using a large spoon, make the servings as big or small as you like.

4 Heat a medium sauté pan over medium heat, then add in the ghee or cooking oil.

5 Place the arepas in, cooking each side for 5 minutes. If anything feels soft, cook them for a bit longer.

6 Eat immediately. Serve plain, or with an egg or other spread on top.

7 Store in the refrigerator for later use.

AREPAS WITH MINCED AVOCADO CHICKEN

In Colombia, you'll find arepas filled with all sorts of goodness: cheese and corn, chicken and beans, whatever your heart desires.

I played around with putting minced chicken inside arepas, and you can totally do the same. For the same good taste and a little less work, you could also make the arepas and just put a dollop of minced chicken on top.

Though the recipe calls for bone-in and skin-on chicken, you can definitely do this with boneless and skinless, but my reasoning is that chicken cooked with the skin on has a bit more flavor and healthy fat, provided that you are buying good-quality chicken. Cooking with the skin side up helps to prevent the chicken from drying out too much. Save the bones to make bone broth.

Makes 4 servings

2 bone-in, skin-on chicken breasts (you can also buy a cooked rotisserie chicken)

½ teaspoon sea salt

¼ cup grated cheese (optional; omit for dairy free)

1 avocado

salt and pepper, to taste

1 Preheat the oven to 375°F.

2 Prepare a baking sheet with a sheet of parchment paper on top to help with clean up.

3 Sprinkle salt on both sides of the chicken breast, then place on the parchment paper skin-side up.

4 Bake in the oven for 30 minutes, remove, and allow to cool for 10 to 15 minutes.

5 Remove skin (you can give it to someone else to eat if it's hard for you to digest).

6 Pull the meat off of the bone and place it in a blender. Blend until chicken pieces are as small as possible. Add cheese, if using.

7 Place the chicken pieces in a large mixing bowl. Scoop out the avocado and add it to the bowl.

8 Using a fork, mash the avocado and mix it well with the chicken.

9 Taste. Add salt and pepper if needed.

10 Place a little scoop on top of Basic Arepas (page 110) as a small meal.

Directions for Arepas Stuffed with Minced Chicken

1 Follow steps 1 and 2 in the Basic Arepas recipe and make the Minced Chicken without the avocado.

2 Heat a large sauté pan over medium heat.

3 Add a generous amount of cooking oil.

4 Before handling the arepa mix, it's easier if you wet your hands with water first.

5 Take a large spoonful of arepa mix and flatten it in your palm. Place a smaller amount of minced chicken in your palm and flatten it.

6 Take another spoonful of arepa mix and place it over top. Join the arepa mix together so that it completely surrounds the chicken. Place in pan.

7 Repeat, adding the arepas to the pan until it is full.

8 Cook each side for roughly 5 minutes.

9 Allow to cool for a bit and enjoy! You can freeze these for later enjoyment.

CHARD AND RED PEPPER EGG BITES

Eggs are a nutritious bite-size package—they contain all the nutrition that a growing chicken needs. Plus, the protein in eggs is extremely bioavailable, which means you can absorb them easily. Some people are sensitive to them, but if you can handle them, they pack in a lot of nutrition.

These egg bites include pureed Swiss chard and red peppers, both extremely nutritious on their own. Swiss chard is a great source of carotenes and vitamins C, E, and K. Red peppers, and bell peppers in general, are extremely nutrient dense. They have abundant amounts of vitamin C, thiamine, folic acid, vitamin B6, and the antioxidant lycopene.

You could theoretically mix and match the veggies that you puree into these egg bites. Play around a bit.

Makes 12 bites

8 eggs

1 bunch Swiss chard leaves (roughly 7 large leaves), pulled from stems

1 large red bell pepper, deseeded and cut into pieces

1 teaspoon salt, plus more to top before baking

Minced Chicken without the avocado, recipe on page 111 (optional)

1 Crack the 8 eggs into a blender and add in the chard, red pepper, and 1 teaspoon salt.

2 Blend until smooth.

3 Preheat the oven to 350°F.

4 Prepare a muffin tin pan with baking cups. Pour the mixture evenly into the cups.

5 If using Minced Chicken, sprinkle chicken onto the tops of the baking cups.

6 Taking a palm full of sea salt, sprinkle each egg bite with a few grains of salt.

7 Bake for 12 minutes.

8 Allow to cool, and enjoy.

CHAWAN MUSHI (STEAMED EGG)

This steamed egg in a cup has an almost light custard-like consistency that, to me, is really fun to eat. It's a classic Japanese dish that normally includes chicken, shrimp, and some mushrooms and onions inside. We've taken away all of those fixings, but if you find that you want to experiment and add any cooked veggies to this egg mixture, please do!

Makes 2 servings

2 eggs

1 cup broth

¼ teaspoon salt or soy sauce

1 Crack the eggs into a small mixing bowl and whisk until mixed.

2 Add in the broth and salt or soy sauce. Mix thoroughly.

3 Divide the mixture between two small bowls that can be heated.

4 Fill the bottom of a large saucepan with half an inch of water.

5 Place the steamer basket in the saucepan, or simply use a heat-resistant plate that almost covers the bottom of the saucepan.

6 Place bowls into steamer.

7 Place over medium heat and bring to a simmer.

8 Simmer for 10 minutes.

9 Be careful taking bowls out, and allow to cool slightly.

10 Enjoy!

SAAG ALOO

Saag aloo literally means spinach and potatoes, and is a common Indian dish from the region of Punjab. I chose to put the dish in this book because it's flavorful and uses basic foods that many GPers do well with. You could also blend this pretty easily and add a bit of broth or water to make it into a soup.

Again, try this as a basic recipe, and if you do well with potatoes and spinach, you can add some of the spices to make it a little more flavorful. These directions call for peeling and cubing the potatoes before you parboil them, but you can also boil them whole with the skins until you can stick a fork through. Let them cool a bit, and then the skins should easily come off. Then you can slice them and put them in the pan. Feel free to substitute ghee for coconut oil.

Makes 4 servings

BASIC INGREDIENTS

2 large potatoes, peeled and cubed

1 quart filtered water

1 tablespoon coconut oil

1 bunch spinach, roughly chopped

½ teaspoon salt, or more to taste

FOR VARIATION

1 sliced onion (high FODMAP)

1 teaspoon turmeric

1 teaspoon garam masala

Directions with Basic Ingredients:

1 Place potatoes in a medium saucepan, cover the cubes with filtered water, and put on medium heat. Cover.

2 Bring to a boil and let simmer for 8 to 10 minutes until you can stick a fork through and the potato is soft. It doesn't need to be completely cooked. Strain.

3 Heat a large sauté pan over medium heat. Add the ghee or coconut oil and the and potatoes. Stir.

4 Add the spinach and stir. Replace the cover.

5 Cook until the spinach and potatoes are soft.

6 Sprinkle with salt. Taste. Add more salt if needed.

Directions for High-FODMAP Variation

1 Repeat steps 1 to 3 above.

2 Heat up large sauté pan over medium heat. Add the ghee or coconut oil, and, if using, the onions. Lower the heat.

3 Add the turmeric and garam masala and mix in with onions and ghee.

4 Cook for roughly 2 to 3 minutes.

5 Add the strained potatoes and spinach. Cover and cook until potatoes are soft.

6 Turn off the heat. Sprinkle with salt. Taste and add more salt if needed.

TURKEY BURGERS

Turkey tends to be lower in fat than other ground meats, so it can be a better option if you don't digest fat well. Most of the fat in turkey lies in the skin. Dark meat has more fat than breast meat, so depending on how you digest fats, you might want to choose one over the other. Turkey is a good source of protein, minerals, B vitamins, and especially the amino acid tryptophan, which is an important building block of serotonin.

This recipe adds liver to your hamburger patties to increase nutrients. It's an easy way to sneak in more nutrients.

In any burger, you can always add more things that agree with you. You have the option of adding some pureed vegetables. Feel free to experiment. The great thing about these patties is that you can freeze them individually and bring them out when you are ready to eat one.

Makes roughly 10 (3-inch-wide) patties

BASIC INGREDIENTS

2 tablespoons hot water

1 teaspoon gelatin

1 pound ground turkey

2 tablespoons pureed liver

¾ teaspoon sea salt

2 tablespoons cooking oil

FOR HIGH-FODMAP VARIATION

½ onion, roughly chopped

2 cloves garlic, roughly chopped

2 medium carrots, roughly chopped

½ medium red onion, roughly chopped

1 Mix the hot water and gelatin in stirring cup until well dissolved.

2 In a large mixing bowl, place in the ground turkey, liver, salt, and gelatin mixture.

3 Either using a fork or your hands, mix thoroughly.

4 Wash your hands after mixing.

5 Heat a large sauté pan over medium heat until warm.

6 Add one tablespoon of cooking oil.

7 Using your hands, form 3-inch by ¼-inch-patties, and place them in the pan. Cook each side for approximately 4 minutes. Add remaining cooking oil, and cook until all of the mixture is used.

8 Eat directly, or freeze individually by putting them on a plate in the freezer for at least 5 hours. Then place in an airtight container and freeze.

High-FODMAP Variation

1 Sauté any optional ingredients you are using until well cooked.

2 Using an immersion blender, blend them until smooth.

3 Mix the hot water and gelatin in stirring cup until well dissolved.

4 In a large mixing bowl, place in the ground turkey, liver, salt, gelatin mixture, and any pureed vegetables.

5 Follow remaining steps from recipe above.

ASIAN-STYLE GROUND PORK

I've heard varying opinions from GPers on ground meats. Sometimes they are tolerated, so I wanted to include a few ways to cook them. Ground meat is a nice way to buy high-quality meat and keep it economical. Plus, you can freeze what you make in single servings for days when you don't feel like cooking. You can make this dish on the stovetop in about 45 minutes, or you can leave all ingredients in the slow cooker for 6 hours or overnight.

Makes 6 to 8 servings

1 pound pastured ground pork

¾ cup water or bone broth

2 tablespoons tamari

1 teaspoon sesame oil

½ teaspoon ginger, minced, or in large chunks (optional)

2 tablespoons rice wine or mirin (optional)

1 tablespoon gelatin

salt, to taste

1 Place the ground pork in a large, lidded sauté pan over medium heat. Using a fork, separate the pieces until the entire pan is covered. Add the water or bone broth and stir occasionally.

2 Stir in the tamari, sesame oil, and ginger and rice wine or mirin, if using.

3 Cover with a lid and bring heat down to a simmer.

4 Simmer for 30 to 45 minutes. After 30 minutes taste and see if it's as tender as you like. The longer you cook it the more tender it gets, and perhaps the easier for you to digest.

5 Sprinkle in the gelatin and mix thoroughly. Taste, and add salt as needed.

6 Eat with rice, congee, or on its own.

MISO-GLAZED DOVER SOLE GF DF LOW FOD MAP

Fish is a lighter protein that can work better for some GPers. You can try this recipe plain as well, with just lemon and salt as a garnish. If you need to throw something together for dinner, this dish is something that takes minimal effort and packs a great amount of flavor. Plus, dover sole is on the Monterey Bay Aquarium Seafood Watch list of sustainable seafood. Seafood Watch is an app and website that you can look on to find more sustainably caught and healthy seafood. I highly recommend it.

Makes 4 servings

1 pound dover sole, sliced

2 tablespoons white miso

2 tablespoons filtered water

lemon (optional)

1 Preheat the oven to 350°F.

2 Line a cookie sheet or baking pan with parchment.

3 In a small bowl, mix the miso and water together until blended. Pour onto a small plate.

4 Coat fish slices with the miso mixture on both side, and place on the cooking sheet. Transfer to oven.

5 Bake thin slices for 6 to 7 minutes; thicker slices for 8 to 9 minutes. If you have mixed thicknesses, you may want to remove slices that are thinner when they are done.

6 Garnish with fresh lemon juice, if desired, and serve with a grain and a veggie.

BAKED SALMON

Salmon is one of the easiest things to make and is extremely high in omega-3 fatty acids, which are essential for brain function and heart health. It's also extremely high in selenium, which is important for prostate health and thyroid function.

Wild Alaskan salmon is the salmon of choice. It's sustainable and is the least contaminated among fish in general. If you cannot find fresh or frozen Alaskan salmon, canned salmon is the next best choice.

Makes 2 servings

1 (6- to 8-inch) salmon fillet

sprinkle sea salt

fresh or dry rosemary sprigs (optional)

lemon slices (optional)

1 Preheat the oven to 375°F.

2 Sprinkle both sides of the salmon fillet with salt.

3 Place the salmon fillet on a baking pan. Add rosemary sprigs or lemon slices on top, if using.

4 Bake for roughly 10 minutes and check. You can use a fork to see if pieces flake off. It's OK if the salmon is slightly translucent in the middle.

5 Remove from the oven and let rest for 5 minutes. Garnish with additional lemon slices, and serve.

SALMON STEW

GF DF LOW FOD MAP

I was introduced to this recipe during a cooking series I ran with a few colleagues. It was a hit! It has few ingredients and is incredibly delicious. The heartiness of the potatoes goes well with the lightness of the salmon.

Often, a great way to make a great fish broth is to buy fish heads at the store. They are usually discarded, and are extremely affordable. Fish heads are a powerhouse of nutrition and full of iodine, which is necessary for thyroid health. Remember that fish broth only needs a short simmering; 20 minutes to one hour and done. For a high-FODMAP variation, sauté onions and leeks before adding liquid. If you can tolerate cow's milk, use cream instead of coconut milk.

Serves 4

1 tablespoon butter or coconut oil

3 cups water, chicken broth, or fish broth

¾ pound potatoes, peeled and cubed

1 bay leaf

¾ cup coconut milk

¾ pound salmon fillet, skinned, de-boned, and cut into small chunks

salt and pepper, to taste

1 Heat a large stockpot over medium heat until warm.

2 Add the butter or coconut oil.

3 Add water or broth.

4 Add cubed potatoes and bay leaf, and let simmer for 15 minutes until soft.

5 Add cream or coconut milk, and then add fish.

6 Simmer for another 5 minutes.

7 Add salt and pepper.

SMALL BITES

CREAMED PARSNIPS WITH PARSLEY

`GF` `DF` `LOW FOD MAP`

I first tried this recipe after I had a tooth pulled, and I was trying to eat soft and nutrient-dense foods. My friend Amaya suggested I eat creamed parsnips. Parsnips are a root vegetable and look much like a carrot, but the texture is slightly different. They are high in fiber, folate, vitamin C, and potassium. I find them to be rather sweet when roasted. If you can tolerate garlic, roast one or two cloves along with the parsnips for a delicious, yet high-FODMAP, addition. Puree garlic with the parsnips for extra flavor. Use ghee or butter in place of coconut milk if you can tolerate dairy.

Makes 4 servings

5 to 6 medium parsnips, peeled if skins look old

¼ to ½ cup broth or filtered water

1 large pat coconut oil

1 handful fresh parsley

salt and pepper, to taste

1 Preheat the oven to 375°F. On a large baking pan, place parsnips with the skin on.

2 Bake for 30 to 40 minutes, until you can stick a fork through the parsnips easily.

3 Place the parsnips in a medium mixing bowl.

4 Using a blender or an immersion blender, add the broth and butter, and blend until smooth. Add more liquid if desired.

5 Add the parsley and a pinch of salt and pepper, and blend again. Taste. Experiment until you find the right taste for you.

BABA GANOUSH

Baba ganoush is a Lebanese dish of roasted eggplant that is very simple to make and pretty darn delicious. Typically, it's made with tahini and garlic. They are optional in this recipe, but if they work for you, then add them and enjoy what they bring to the dish.

Eggplant is in season over the summer months and is in the family of nightshade plants that include potatoes, peppers, and tomatoes. It is a good source of minerals and B vitamins. This recipe takes the skin off to reduce fiber content, but as you play around with foods and if you have a powerful blender, you could try keeping a bit of the skin as many nutrients and antioxidants are there. You could also increase or decrease the amount of olive oil to fit your needs. For a more traditional (but high-FODMAP) recipe, include 2 tablespoons of tahini and 1 clove of garlic in step 7.

Makes 8 small servings

2 globe eggplants

¼ cup broth

1 tablespoon extra-virgin olive oil

¼ teaspoon sea salt, plus more to taste

1 teaspoon lemon juice

1 Preheat the oven to 375°F.

2 Take a fork and poke a few holes in the eggplant.

3 Place on a baking sheet or pan.

4 Bake for 15 to 20 minutes or until skin turns wrinkly.

5 Remove from the oven and allow to cool for 10 to 15 minutes.

6 Scrape out eggplant with a spoon and place in blender or mixing bowl.

7 Add the broth, olive oil, sea salt, and lemon juice.

8 Blend together using blender or immersion blender.

9 Taste. Add more sea salt if necessary.

KOHLRABI MASH

Kohlrabi is part of the cabbage family, and when cooked, has a sweet and delicate flavor and texture. It is helpful for balancing blood sugar, and is an excellent source of vitamin C and potassium. Look for smaller bulbs when buying, as the smaller they are, the sweeter they will be.

Makes 4 servings

6 medium bulbs kohlrabi, leaves removed

1 medium potato

1 quart filtered water

1 tablespoon butter or coconut oil

¼ cup broth

salt, to taste

1 Place kohlrabi and potato in a medium pot. Cover with water.

2 Over medium heat, bring to a boil. Boil for roughly 20 minutes or until you can stick a fork through easily.

3 Remove from pot and allow to cool slightly.

4 Using a knife, cut the outer skin off of the kohlrabi. Use your fingers to peel the skin off the potato.

5 The bottom of the kohlrabi is a bit tougher, so take a larger slice out and roughly chop the kohlrabi into large chunks (smaller if you are putting them into a blender).

6 Blend the kohlrabi and potato in a blender, or with an immersion blender, with butter/oil and a splash of broth.

7 Add remaining broth for a smoother consistency.

8 Salt to taste, blend, taste, and add more salt if necessary.

ROASTED RED BELL PEPPERS

Red bell peppers are a tasty way to get some great nutrients in. High in vitamin C and full of antioxidants, when roasted they have a sweeter, distinct taste that you can use in a number of ways. You can eat them on their own, blend them into Turkey Burgers (page 117), or mix them in with any of the soup purees to add a little red pepper flavor.

Makes 4 to 6 servings

4 medium red bell peppers, tops and seeds removed

1 Preheat the oven to 450°F.

2 Spread parchment paper over a baking sheet.

3 Lay each pepper skin side up.

4 Bake for roughly 25 minutes, until skins are slightly charred and wrinkly.

5 Remove from baking sheet and allow to cool for 20 minutes.

6 Remove skins and discard.

7 Eat with a pinch of salt or splash of extra-virgin olive oil.

8 If saving, place in airtight container in fridge or freezer for later use.

SWEET POTATO MASH

GF DF

Sweet potatoes are not related at all to the potato family, and are native to Central and South America. They are sweet, satisfying, and easy to bake. They are extremely nutrient dense. High in carotenes, vitamin C, and manganese, they are also anti-inflammatory and good for blood sugar regulation. There are many different types, from the bright orange-flesh Beauregards that are common in the US to purple-flesh and white-flesh types. Try them all! Sweet potatoes are technically not low fiber nor low FODMAP, so try a small amount to see if it agrees with you.

Makes 2 servings

1 large sweet potato

1/4 cup any milk, such as coconut or almond, or filtered water

1/16 teaspoon sea salt

1 teaspoon coconut oil

1/16 teaspoon cinnamon

1 Preheat the oven to 375ºF.

2 Using a fork, perforate the skin all around the sweet potato. This will help to release steam while it is roasting.

3 Arrange on a roasting pan or baking sheet and roast in the oven for roughly 45 minutes. When a fork slides through effortlessly, it's done.

4 Slice open and scoop out the contents into large bowl. Add liquid or milk, and mash thoroughly.

5 Add the sea salt, coconut oil, and cinnamon.

6 Taste and adjust accordingly.

LIVER PUREE

Liver, the storehouse for many minerals and vitamins, is one of the most nutrient-dense parts of an animal that we can consume. When we eat the liver of a healthy animal, we get those nutrients in a compact form. This simple liver puree can be eaten on its own or mixed in with Turkey Burgers (page 117) or the Asian-Style Ground Pork (page 119) for extra nutrient density. I learned this trick from working at Three Stone Hearth, a kitchen in Berkeley that prepares food according to the philosophy of Weston A. Price and tries to be as nutrient dense as possible. If the liver flavor is too strong for you, this is a way to hide and blend the flavors in something else.

You can spread this onto gluten-free crackers or cucumbers that are peeled and deseeded.

Makes 8 servings

1 tablespoon cooking oil

1 pound liver

salt and pepper, to taste

1 Heat a large sauté pan over medium heat until warm.

2 Add the cooking oil.

3 Add the liver and cook until the insides are still slightly pink.

4 Transfer to a medium mixing bowl, and using an immersion blender, blend until smooth. Add salt and pepper.

5 Enjoy as a spread, or freeze for use in other recipes.

6 To freeze, place into ice cube trays and freeze for a minimum of five hours. Remove from tray and place in an airtight container.

PÃO DE QUEIJO (BRAZILIAN CHEESE BREAD)

Pão de queijo translates into cheese bread, which means that this recipe is not dairy free. If you can handle dairy, these little snacks are spongy, airy treats that cook quickly and reheat well. They provide protein and calories, but in terms of nutrient density, these are a once-in-awhile treat. Enjoy!

Makes 9 small puffs

4 tablespoons butter

3 tablespoons cow's milk

2 tablespoons plus 1 teaspoon filtered water

½ teaspoon sea salt

1 cup tapioca flour

½ teaspoon baking soda

1 egg

1 cup grated cheese (any kind)

1 Preheat oven to 375°F.

2 Prepare a baking sheet by spreading a piece of parchment paper on top. Set aside.

3 Pour butter, milk, water, and salt into a medium saucepan. Bring to a boil and turn off heat.

4 Place the tapioca flour in a large bowl and pour in the butter and milk/water mixture.

5 Using a spoon, mix thoroughly and allow to sit for 10 to 15 minutes.

6 Rub a little olive oil or butter onto your hands.

7 Add the baking soda, egg, and cheese. Mix thoroughly with your hands. Optionally, you can mix and knead the dough for up to 10 minutes. This helps get more air in and will create a more puffed-up bread.

8 Place ¼-cup-size balls on the sheet.

9 Bake for 15 to 20 minutes or until tops are golden brown.

10 Eat immediately.

SWEET TREATS

The fact that this chapter is named "treats" is an important idea. You want to "treat" things that contain sweeteners as once-in-a-while indulgences. If you find that you can tolerate the muffins in this section well, I would suggest lowering the amount of sweetener if you are eating them more regularly. Be mindful, however, that you should be looking for variety in the diet, and since some of the following treats are made with gluten-free flours, too much can start to create imbalances in the body. I would start making any of the muffin recipes as mini muffins, and see how your body does.

BLUEBERRY ALMOND MUFFINS

You can buy almond flour or almond meal to bake with, but I would start with almond flour to see how you react to it, and then experiment with almond meal. It will be worth trying both kinds to see which one you deal with better. Note: almond flour/meal in small amounts can be low FODMAP, but having too much might backfire on you.

Almond creates a gluten free-flour that is low in fiber; ¼ cup of uncooked almond flour (which is the serving size of one of these muffins) contains just 3 grams of dietary fiber. Each mini muffin will contain roughly ⅛ cup of almond flour, so each serving should have around 1½ grams of dietary fiber from the almond flour.

Makes 8 mini muffins

2 eggs

½ ripe banana

1 tablespoon plus 1 teaspoon coconut oil, melted

½ teaspoon apple cider vinegar

1 tablespoon honey or maple syrup

1 cup almond flour

⅛ teaspoon sea salt

¼ teaspoon baking soda

¼ teaspoon baking powder (optional, for fluffier muffins)

¾ cup blueberries

1 Preheat the oven to 350°F and place mini muffin cups in a mini muffin tin.

2 In a large mixing bowl, crack the eggs and place in the banana, melted coconut oil, apple cider vinegar, and sweetener.

3 Mash and mix well with a fork, or use an immersion blender to blend until smooth.

4 Add the almond meal, salt, baking soda, and baking powder, if using.

5 Mix until thoroughly incorporated

6 Add blueberries, and with a spatula, gently fold them in.

7 Spoon ¼ cup of the mixture into each muffin tin.

8 Bake for 15 to 20 minutes until done.

CHOCOLATE CHIP ALMOND MUFFINS

Cocoa powder is full of antioxidants and can be stimulating for some people. Depending on the person, it can be too stimulating, so always use cocoa powder and chocolate with mindfulness. You will use almond meal again for these muffins and can make them with a few base ingredients. Then, if you handle these well, you can add some coconut oil, cinnamon, and vanilla.

Makes 8 mini muffins

2 eggs

1 banana

1 tablespoon plus 1 teaspoon coconut oil, melted (optional)

½ teaspoon vanilla (optional)

1 cup almond meal

4 tablespoons cocoa powder

¼ teaspoon baking soda

¼ teaspoon baking powder

⅛ teaspoon sea salt

½ teaspoon cinnamon (optional)

½ cup dark/bittersweet chocolate chips

1 Preheat the oven to 350°F and place mini muffin cups in a mini muffin tin.

2 In a large mixing bowl, crack the eggs and place in the banana, and add melted coconut oil and vanilla, if using.

3 Mash and mix well with a fork, or, using an immersion blender, blend until smooth.

4 Add the almond meal, cocoa powder, baking soda, baking powder, cinnamon (if using), and salt. Mix well with a spatula.

5 Mix in the chocolate chips.

6 Put a heaping tablespoon of muffin batter into each mini muffin tin.

7 Bake for 10 to 13 minutes.

AVOCADO KEY LIME PUDDING

GF DF

Avocado makes a wonderful, creamy pudding. This is the filling that I make for a key lime pie that goes into the freezer to harden; I also like it creamy and smooth as a pudding. It's satisfying and fun to eat.

Makes 2 servings

2 ripe medium avocados

4 teaspoons honey

1 pinch salt

4 teaspoons lime juice

2 tablespoons coconut oil (optional, to add a little more fat)

1 Cut each avocado in half and spoon the contents into a food processor or large mixing bowl. Add the honey, salt, lime juice, and coconut oil, if using.

2 Blend in the food processor or using an immersion blender until smooth.

3 Place into bowls and enjoy!

AVOCADO CHOCOLATE PUDDING

Makes 4 servings

3 avocados

2 to 3 tablespoons cocoa powder

½ cup coconut milk or almond milk (optional)

¼ cup maple syrup, plus more to taste

1 teaspoon ground cinnamon (optional)

⅛ teaspoon sea salt

1 Using a spoon, scoop the avocado into a large mixing bowl.

2 Add the cocoa powder, coconut or almond milk (if using), maple syrup, cinnamon (if using), and sea salt.

3 Using an immersion blender or fork, blend all of the ingredients together until smooth.

4 Taste. Add more of any ingredient if necessary.

5 Serve on its own or as a frosting for muffins.

SOOTHING SWEETENED JELLIES

The sweetened gelatin (Jell-O) that you find in stores and at your average party might be nostalgic, but it's full of artificial ingredients. What gives these jellies their healing abilities and texture is gelatin, the culinary term for collagen, of which there are many benefits. It pretty much holds us together. It gives our skin its strength and suppleness, and is an integral part of our bones, joints, and connective tissue. It's healing to the gut and considered to be a digestive aid. This recipe is inspired by my apprenticeship at Three Stone Hearth. They made amazing gelatines of many flavors. Thanks, Three Stone!

Makes 4 servings

1 cup fruit juice (any kind)

1 cup water

2 tablespoons coconut sugar or palm sugar

4 teaspoons gelatin

1 Before you start, set up 4 cup-size containers. I like half-pint mason jars that you can pour the mixture directly into.

2 In a medium saucepan, heat the juice, water, and sugar over medium heat until it starts to simmer. Turn off the heat.

3 Using an immersion blender or whisk, slowly add the gelatin and blend/whisk until fully blended.

4 Pour into jars; each jar will be half filled. Close the lids, and if you'd like to enjoy them sooner rather than later, place in the freezer for 20 minutes until solid. Otherwise, place in the fridge to enjoy after roughly 6 hours.

CHOCOLATE BANANA ICE CREAM

Bananas are pretty incredible. They have such an interesting consistency that lends smoothness to smoothies and holds baked goods together. Another fun fact: they make great ice cream. If you do well with cocoa powder, then make it chocolate. You could also play around by adding other tolerated ingredients to this if you like; peanut butter or almond butter make a nice addition.

Bananas themselves are actually considered a berry. (Shout out to Daniel Gritzer at seriouseats.com for that tidbit.) They are grown in tropical areas and shipped to the US.

Bananas provide good minerals, and as they ripen, the more the starches will turn into sugars. Do not overeat them for this reason.

Sometimes I buy bananas but don't get a chance to eat them before they get too ripe. So, I'll follow step one of the recipe and just freeze them until I'm ready to make ice cream.

Makes 2 servings

2 ripe bananas

1 tablespoon cocoa powder

1 pinch salt

1 tablespoon nut butter, optional

1 Peel the bananas and roughly chop them into slices. Place them in an airtight container and freeze for a minimum of 2 hours.

2 Place the bananas, cocoa powder, and salt in a food processor or strong blender. You may add any additional ingredients here (nut butter, for example).

3 Blend until smooth.

4 Serve as is, or place back in freezer to harden before enjoying.

BEVERAGES

You may be able to handle liquids better than solids, and if so, then the next section is great for you. Beverages are a great way to get in hydration, and at the same time, more nutrients. Give them a try!

HOMEMADE ELECTROLYTE DRINK `GF` `DF` `LOW FOD MAP`

Factory-made electrolyte drinks like Pedialyte or Gatorade are often recommended for dehydration; they mainly provide electrolytes to the body. However, these store-bought drinks are also filled with many artificial ingredients. Instead, you want to make sure you keep what is going on inside your body as clean as possible. You can make your own hydrating beverage easily with three basic ingredients. You can add a splash of juice or herbal tea.

Makes 4 servings

2 tablespoons maple syrup or honey

1 quart filtered water, room temperature or slightly warm

½ teaspoon sea salt

1 Mix maple syrup, filtered water, and sea salt together in a glass jar.

2 Stir until dissolved.

3 Drink!

DIY ALMOND MILK

I've talked with a few gastroparesis patients who are lactose intolerant, and almond milk can be a great substitute (you can also sub in just about any other nut—hazelnut is delicious as well). I generally counsel people to try making their own almond milk for a few reasons. One is that it is *delicious*, and the other is that store-bought almond milks can have a lot of artificial additives. You can use this as a base for smoothies, or just enjoy a glass on its own.

Makes 1 quart

1 cup almonds, soaked overnight

4 cups filtered water

1 tablespoon maple syrup

¼ teaspoon vanilla

¹⁄₁₆ teaspoon sea salt

½ teaspoon cinnamon

1 Place soaked almonds and water in a blender and blend.

2 Using a clean dish towel or finely meshed sieve, strain into a separate container.

3 Set almond pulp aside for use in pancakes or baking.

4 Rinse blender and place strained almond milk back into blender with maple syrup, vanilla, sea salt, and cinnamon. Blend.

5 Taste and adjust seasonings.

6 Enjoy immediately or store in fridge for 3 to 4 days.

GINGER CINNAMON TEA

Ginger is great for nausea and inflammation, among other things. Cinnamon is wonderful for regulating blood sugar and helping to fix a sweet craving. I like this tea because it is incredibly easy to make, and if you like the spiciness of ginger, you can leave it in for longer and store the tea with the ginger pieces as well.

Makes 4 servings

1 quart filtered water

1 claw ginger

1 stick cinnamon

1 tablespoon honey

1 Slice ginger into large chunks.

2 In a medium saucepan, place the water, ginger, and cinnamon over medium to high heat until the water starts boil.

3 Lower heat, cover, and simmer for 10 to 15 minutes. Turn off heat.

4 Stir in the honey.

5 Drink immediately or leave tea covered to steep for longer. Wait until contents have cooled and pour entire contents into a jar to store in the fridge for later use.

6 If you do not want the tea too spicy, you can take out the ginger pieces when you want. Taste as you go.

MEXICAN HOT CHOCOLATE `GF` `DF` `LOW FOD MAP`

Plain cocoa powder is full of antioxidants and oh so rich and satisfying. This is something that I use to treat myself on a cold winter day.

Makes 1 serving

1 cup filtered water, almond milk, or coconut milk

1 tablespoon cocoa powder

pinch ground cinnamon

pinch cayenne pepper

pinch sea salt

1 teaspoon maple syrup

1 Heat the water or milk in a small saucepan over a low flame.

2 When warm, add the cocoa powder, cinnamon, cayenne pepper, sea salt, and maple syrup.

3 Taste. Add more of any ingredient as desired.

TURMERIC GINGER ALMOND MILK

Turmeric and ginger are two inflammation-fighting roots that are great to consume regularly. Turmeric and ginger look very similar and have really distinct and strong flavors. Curcumin is the compound in turmeric that gives it the beautiful orange color it's known for and is responsible for the anti-inflammatory effects. Turmeric is also looked at as being beneficial for preventing heart disease and cancer.

You can buy both of these roots powdered, and you'll have to give the powdered herbs a try if you cannot find fresh turmeric and ginger roots. Or, if you can find dried root, it would be a better idea so that you can simmer the roots and take them out before enjoying.

Makes 4 servings

1 small claw fresh ginger, 1 tablespoon dried ginger root, or 1 teaspoon powdered ginger

1 small claw fresh turmeric, 1 tablespoon dried turmeric root, or 1 teaspoon powdered ginger

1 quart almond milk, coconut milk, or any alternative milk

2 tablespoons honey

pinch salt

1 If using fresh roots, slice into large chunks.

2 Place milk of choice and fresh or dried turmeric and ginger in a medium saucepan.

3 Simmer on low, covered, for 15 minutes.

4 Turn off the heat and steep for as long as you like. The longer you allow the roots to steep, the more flavor they will have. Adjust to your taste.

5 Stir in the honey and salt.

6 Enjoy!

SUMMER FRUIT AND MINT YOGURT LASSI

Lassis are a traditional yogurt drink from India. At restaurants, they're frequently prepared with mango and are usually very, very sweet. If you are trying to avoid dairy, then this may not be the best recipe for you. This recipe uses yogurt or kefir, which are two ways to consume fermented foods. Fermented foods provide a good dose of beneficial bacteria, which are helpful for metabolism, digestion, keeping bad bacteria and yeasts in check, and immune system function. Along with eating a whole foods diet, eating fermented foods is helpful to keep populations diverse and strong.

I like this recipe because it uses the natural sweetness of ripe summer fruits, adds a bit of mint, and has a nice tangy taste from the yogurt. The lime adds another beautiful dimension. Try this on hot summer day, and share with friends!

Makes 4 servings

2 cups seedless watermelon or 1 large, ripe peach

1/4 cup lightly packed mint

1 cup whole milk plain yogurt or plain kefir

$\frac{1}{16}$ teaspoon (roughly a pinch) salt

juice 1 lime

sprig mint, to garnish

Place all of the ingredients in a blender. Blend and serve with a sprig of mint.

JUICED JICAMA

Jicama is a root vegetable native to Mexico and Central America. It's a good source of potassium and vitamin C, and has a high water content that makes it great to juice.

If you have a juicer, this is a great time to use it. However, I simply use a clean dish towel or nut milk bag to strain the pulp out. You could also use a fine sieve. This recipe is *perfectly* delicious on its own, but you can include a hint of lime to add a little extra.

Makes 2 servings

1 medium jicama, peeled and cut 1 inch thick

¼ cup filtered water

pinch salt

squeeze lime (optional)

1 Place jicama and water in a powerful blender. Blend.

2 Take a jar and place funnel on top.

3 Using a clean dish towel, fine sieve, or nut milk bag, pour jicama and water mixture into cloth and squeeze juice out into the jar.

4 Squeeze thoroughly.

5 Add pinch of salt and lime juice, if using.

6 Discard pulp and enjoy immediately, or refrigerate for later use.

Chapter 7
HOLISTIC VIEW OF DISEASE

It's impossible to talk about a holistic view of disease without talking about a holistic view of health. One defines the other. Each of us is trying to find ease, a state of repose, a state of health. If you look at the word disease, you can break it up into *dis* and *ease*. Something or things are pulling us out of ease.

I have already discussed a large portion of what consists of holistic health. Reducing stress, movement, nourishing foods, sleep, community—I won't expand on those sections here, but it *is* important to see the overlap. When you look at how to heal, you look at how to bring into balance many different aspects.

Remember how Judith Aston, the woman who I'm learning more about alignment and movement from, describes neutral (page 31). I love her definition because it fits so well with what holistic health means to me: Being in the least possible stress and providing the most support for our bodies, both mentally and physically. These elements of health are not meant to be focused on all at once. Especially since there are going to be days when your symptoms might be all-encompassing, and those days are not going to be easy.

On those days, how can you make decisions that best support how you are feeling?

Let's look at this with an open mind, and with a mind that looks into the future. It's time to talk about some basic tenets of holistic health.

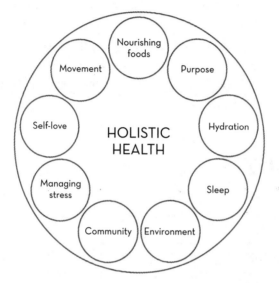

Your goal is to try and bring these aspects into balance so that on days that you are out of balance, you can stay closer to center. Our bodies can be very resilient, but if we lack one aspect for too long, it can exacerbate dis-ease. So, the ultimate goal is when you have the space for it, check in and move forward in one of these areas.

We've already discussed a few sections earlier, so let me take a moment to talk about self-love, purpose, and environment in a little more detail.

SELF-LOVE

Self-love can mean a lot of different things, but ultimately, it should answer the question, am I taking care of myself in a loving and compassionate way? Most people sacrifice themselves to work a little longer, to get one more errand done, to take care of that family member, instead of feeding themselves or getting some down time.

As someone who is diagnosed with gastroparesis, it's even *more* important to give yourself plenty of self-love and care. You will get to know your body's patterns, what foods work for you, and what times of the day you feel less symptomatic. Many GP folks find that the mornings are better for them, and symptoms can start to flare at night. Being gentle with your own boundaries and creating a space where you can be kind to yourself (not scheduling anything after 4 p.m., for example) can be helpful.

PURPOSE

Purpose, or you can call it your mission in life, is different for everyone. I personally feel that my life has a purpose, that I was put here to do something positive for the world and to bring joy and positive change into people's lives. Some people know from when they are little what they are called to do, and others don't find it until after they've spent decades searching.

In our discussion of holistic health, and especially for those with chronic illness, it's helpful to ask, what do you want to be healthy for? Why do you want energy? Sometimes focusing on that goal can give you energy where you felt you didn't have any.

My conversation with Tae-Lynn, whose life purpose is to spread more kindness in the world, was an inspiring talk.

Personal Insight
Tae-Lynn, 54, outside of Philadelphia

"I have a couple of painful illnesses, and for anyone who is suffering through any chronic illness, it's really important to take care of your spirit and your mind.

At one point, I had the plan for suicide. I had the pills, I had everything. My kidneys were severely compromised (and still are); I couldn't just take whatever prescription. I couldn't get pregnant, I couldn't have kids, my job was ripped away from me. I was so depressed, I was single, I had been married and divorced, and then I had one of those dark nights, when I heard the voice that told me I was fine as I was.

Finding my purpose really helped bring me out of the spiral. Find your purpose, even if it might not be what you thought it was, but it's a gift there for you to find.

I found my purpose through kindness. Kindness can improve our own health. We are stuck sometimes wallowing in our own problems, but when we volunteer and help other people it can bring us out of it. I became a hospice volunteer and it helped me immensely. Many people tell me they are too sick, but I've been there with my chronic fatigue and fibromyalgia. There's always something that you can do. You can make a phone call from your bed—there are a lot of organizations that need people to do phone calls. I struggled with the first few years, until I had that epiphany that gave me a reason to get out of bed. Just to walk the dogs. People need purpose. Your mood will affect how you feel. It's not a cure, but it's going to affect how you feel, and that has a huge impact. We are all here to help each other in life. I was encouraged to share my story, and since I have, I've been touched by the people who have reached out to me. There's always someone on this journey ahead of you or behind you. You could help someone too."

Find out more about Tae-Lynn on her website: www.60seconds tokindness.com.

Purpose can sometimes be the realization that we are just a small part of a bigger picture. Have you thought about your purpose recently?

ENVIRONMENT

Included in the discussion of environment is what goes on your skin, what you clean your house with, and whether or not your produce is organic. Also, it does help to have clear and uncluttered environment. Sometimes this is where, if someone wants to be of service to you, you could ask them if they could help you tidy up and even get rid of stuff that you don't need.

One book that really swept the holistic circle was *The Life-Changing Magic of Tidying Up*, by Marie Kondo. I saw it transform many people's lives and homes. Another great book is *Clear Your Clutter with Feng Shui*, by Karen Kingston. Karen Kingston talks of unused items simply being stuck energy.

You are looking to make your environment simple and healing. But when items are scattered around gathering dust and being unused, it can feel heavy. Sometimes you may not even notice how heavy your environment feels until you change it.

Try working on a small area at a time, perhaps your nightstand or your desk. You'll feel a sense of pride when you are done, and don't listen to that voice that says, "What if one day I will need this?"

❦

It's time to look at your health through a holistic lens and start at any place, taking small steps when you can. You are really on a journey, not something that can be done in a day, a week, or even a year. This is lifelong, and you always find something to work on as you move forward.

Chapter 8
NUTRITION 101

Each of us receives a surprisingly little amount of nutrition education, which is really a shame, and what I suspect is one of reasons why so many preventable diseases are becoming more and more prevalent. There is a common acronym often heard in holistic nutrition circles, called SAD, which stands for **S**tandard **A**merican **D**iet. As people fall prey to stressful lives, poor nutrition, and overuse of medications, it all becomes a vicious cycle that feeds into a model of treating symptoms and not treating the cause.

It's important for you to know what your body needs to function. Days when you aren't feeling well and are having trouble eating, you should be eating what you can with a knowledge of what you need.

Basically, your body needs energy and building blocks for body structures (which are provided by macronutrients), and chemicals to make things happen in the body (micronutrients). Some things, your body has the ability to make on its own (especially if you are healthy), but others, you must get through the food you eat. So you need to eat.

MACRONUTRIENTS

Let me talk about energy first. You've seen digestion and how complicated the stomach physiology is on its own. The number of things that have to happen as soon as you bite into something for it to be delivered to your cells is astounding. Essentially, you are looking for glucose, a sugar that will feed your cells directly. Where do you get glucose? You get it from carbohydrates, which is one of the three macronutrients that you need larger amounts of in your diet.

Carbohydrates come from vegetables, fruits, starches, and sugars. (Carbohydrates in the form of fruits and vegetables also come packed with colorful antioxidants that are vital in helping the body repair, so remember to eat a rainbow of colors.) Depending on the form they come in, they could be complex, with lots of molecules bound together, or they could be simple, with a very simple molecule chain. This is where you might hear the terms poly-, oligo-, di-, or monosaccharides. The prefixes of these words refer to the number of simple sugars bound together. The body, though, has to transform these more complex sugars into simple sugars to absorb them and convert everything into glucose, which is used by the body for energy.

When you eat simple sugars, like candy, you absorb it rather quickly, which is not something you want. For those of you who have diabetes, this is especially undesirable. You want to absorb things slowly over time. When you eat an excess of simple carbohydrates, your bloodstream is flooded with glucose, which creates blood sugar imbalances and can lead to excess fat storage.

The fat that you store in your body is different from the fat you eat in foods, which is different from the fat that is part of your bodily structures. Let's look more closely at the fat you eat, which is the second macronutrient that you need in larger amounts.

Dietary fat is taken in by the body and broken down into its parts: one glycerol molecule and three fatty acid molecules. Together these are called triglycerides—sound familiar? Fatty acid molecules can be described by length as short-, medium-, or long-chain fatty acids. They can also be described as either saturated or unsaturated. Whether or not a fatty acid is saturated or unsaturated depends on the number of hydrogen atoms bonded to the core carbon atoms. Saturated fatty acids are full of hydrogen atoms, while unsaturated are missing either one hydrogen atom (monounsaturated) or more than one (polyunsaturated). We've all heard these terms before, but they are very rarely explained. For all intents and purposes, foods are filled with a variety of all of these different types of fatty acids, and you should eat a bit of all of them.

The broken-down glycerol and fatty acids enter the liver and your fat cells. In the fat cells, they are put back together into triglycerides and stored for later. When there is a lack of glucose, the body then breaks down triglycerides to be used as energy in the form of fatty acids. You are constantly switching between glucose metabolism and fat metabolism throughout the day.

Fat is also used within the body to make up certain structures. Each cell membrane is created from layers of fat. Cholesterol is also a type of fat that you can get through food, but your body makes a majority of it. Cholesterol is a building block for hormones, such as estrogen and progesterone, and is part of the tissue that surrounds each nerve.

Proteins are the third and final macronutrient, and they also serve as building blocks that you need to maintain your bodily structures. Over "100,000 different proteins are thought to exist in the body."[48] Proteins are made up of different combinations of amino acids. There are roughly 20 naturally occurring amino acids, 12 of which your body can make as long as you are in good health, and eight other amino acids you must get from food—these eight are called essential amino acids. You can also use protein as energy, but it is not the preferred energy source.

---

48 Wynn Kapit, et al., The Physiology Coloring Book, 2nd ed. (San Francisco: Addison Wesley Longman, 2000).

MICRONUTRIENTS

Along with fat, protein, and carbohydrates, the three macronutrients, you also need nutrients called *micro*nutrients. These are the vitamins and minerals that you probably have heard a lot about. The Institute of Medicine created Daily Recommended Intakes (DRIs), which are the levels recommended to a healthy population to prevent disease. (I personally don't like to get too bogged down with numbers and instead choose to focus on eating a variety of foods, which is what this book talks about!)

Vitamins and minerals are responsible for chemical reactions in the body; they are usually paired with an enzyme to either build up or break down components in the body.

Here are the vitamins. They are broken up into two types: fat soluble and water soluble.

Fat-Soluble Vitamins

Can be stored in fat cells and used when needed. They include:

- Vitamin A
- Vitamin D
- Vitamin E
- Vitamin K

Water-Soluble Vitamins

Can only be stored in small amounts, so deficiencies can develop more easily. They include:

- Thiamine (B1)
- Riboflavin (B2)
- Niacin (B3)
- Pantothenic acid (B5)
- Pyridoxine (B6)
- Folic acid
- Vitamin B12
- Biotin
- Choline
- Vitamin C

Each of these vitamins serve specific functions in the body; often, it took diseases to help us understand what exactly they did. Scurvy, which was discovered on long sea voyages, caused gums and joint capsules to bleed, and prevented wounds from healing, was caused by a vitamin C deficiency. Beriberi, which was first documented in Asian countries and caused numbness and eventually paralysis, was discovered to be a thiamine deficiency.

Minerals are also broken up into two categories: major minerals and minor minerals (also called trace minerals).

Major Minerals

We need more than 100 mg daily of these minerals.

- Calcium
- Chloride
- Magnesium
- Phosphorus
- Potassium
- Sodium
- Sulfur

Minor Minerals

- Boron
- Chromium
- Copper
- Iodine
- Iron
- Manganese
- Molybdenum
- Selenium
- Silicon
- Vanadium
- Zinc

Minerals are absorbed with adequate stomach acid, and plants are mineral rich if the soil they are grown in is mineral rich. This is another reason to buy from farms whose priority it is to enrich the soil, which small organic farms aim to do.

Appendix A

LOW-FIBER FOODS

Created from Michael Murray's *The Encyclopedia of Healing Foods*, this appendix lists the amount of fiber for 100 grams of each food. One hundred grams is 3.5 ounces. It's important to note that 100 grams of one food may actually be a lot to eat at one sitting, and 100 grams of another food may be too little. For example, 100 grams of spinach is a lot of spinach to eat, as is 100 grams of almonds. With nuts, about 1 ounce (approximately 1 handful) is a serving size, and the values below reflect 1-ounce amounts. So, these numbers are just to give you an idea of the ratio of fiber in each food. Most likely you will be eating less than 100 grams, so you will probably be taking in less fiber.

Foods that have a star are high in FODMAPs. Also, some of these numbers are for raw vegetables with the skin on, and you will soften and make some fiber more digestible when food is cooked.

An important note about meats: Animal meats do not contain fiber, but you will have to experiment to see which ones work for you. You can try ground meats and pureed meats as options.

FIBER CONTENT OF SELECT FOODS

* indicates high in FODMAPs

VEGETABLES

	fiber per 100 g
Arugula, raw	1.6 g
Asparagus*	1.6 g
Beets, boiled*	2 g
Bell peppers, raw	2 g
Carrots, raw	3 g
Celery, raw	1.7 g
Cucumbers with peel	.8 g
Collard greens, raw	2 g
Kale, raw	2 g
Leeks*	1 g
Mushrooms*	0.6 g
Mustard greens, boiled	2 g
Onions*	1.8 g
Potatoes with skin	2.2 g
Radishes, raw	1.6 g
Spinach, raw	2.7 g
Summer squash, cooked	1.4 g
Sunchokes, raw*	1.6 g
Swiss chard, boiled	2.1 g
Tomatoes, raw	1.1 g
Winter squash, cooked	2.8 g

FRUITS (RAW)

	fiber per 100 g
Apple with skin*	2.7 g
Apricot*	2.4 g
Banana	2.4 g
Blueberries	2.7 g
Cantaloupe	.8 g
Cherries*	2.3 g
Grapes	1 g
Honeydew melon	.6 g
Mango*	1.8 g
Nectarines*	2 g
Orange	2.3 g
Papaya	1.8 g
Peaches*	2 g
Pear*	2.4 g
Pineapple	1.2 g
Plums*	1.5 g
Strawberries	2.3 g
Watermelon*	.5 g

GRAINS

	fiber per 100 g
Brown rice, cooked	1.8 g
Millet, cooked	1.3 g

NUTS

	fiber per 1 oz
Almonds*	3.4 g
Brazil nuts	1.6 g
Cashews*	1.6 g
Chestnuts	1.5 g
Coconut, raw	2.6 g
Flaxseed	8 g
Hazelnuts*	2.8 g
Macadamia nuts	2.3 g
Peanuts	2.3 g
Pecans	2.7 g
Pine nuts	1.3 g
Pistachios*	3 g
Pumpkin seeds	1.1 g
Sesame seeds	3.4 g
Sunflower seeds	3.2 g
Walnuts	2 g

This following lists are adapted from the Monash University FODMAP app, which has very up-to-date information about FODMAPs. It's very user-friendly, with recipes, that you can download to help you shop.

It's interesting to note that the amount of FODMAPs is also based on serving size. Sometimes, for example, 10 almonds is low FODMAP, but 20 is too many. Or, half a cup of coconut water is fine, but 1 cup is too much. So, because you may not be able to eat a lot at once, this may work to your favor in allowing you to eat more foods.

VEGETABLES

Low FODMAP	High FODMAP
Alfalfa sprouts	Artichokes
Arugula	Asparagus
Bamboo shoots	Beets
Bell peppers	Cabbage, fermented
Bok choy	Cassava
Broccoli	Cauliflower
Brussels sprouts	Garlic
Cabbage (not savoy)	Leek bulbs
Carrots	Mushrooms
Chives	Onions
Collard greens	Shallots
Cucumber	Snow peas
Eggplant	Snap peas
Fennel	Sunchokes
Gai lan (Chinese broccoli)	Sweet corn
Ginger	Sweet potatoes
Green beans	Taro
Kabocha squash	Yucca
Kale	
Leek leaves	
Lettuce	
Okra	
Olives	
Onion tops	
Parsnips	
Potatoes	
Radishes	
Seaweed	

FRUITS

Low FODMAP

Bananas
Blueberries
Cantaloupe
Clementines
Dragon fruit
Durian
Grapes
Kiwis
Kumquats
Lemon juice
Lime juice
Mandarins
Oranges
Papayas
Pineapples
Plantains
Raspberries
Rhubarb
Star fruit
Strawberries

High FODMAP

Apples
Apricots
Avocado
Blackberry
Cherries
Figs
Grapefruit
Lychees
Mangoes
Nectarines
Peaches
Pears
Persimmons
Watermelon

Appendix B

INCREASING STOMACH ACID HOLISTICALLY

Stomach acid is a very important aspect of the digestive system and is extremely important for a number of reasons.

- It is your first line of defense for killing pathogens introduced by the food you eat.

- Stomach acid is vital in breaking down the proteins.

- All B vitamins, with the exception of choline, require sufficient stomach acid to be usable.

- Stomach acid is also used in the absorption of many minerals. Minerals that can be depleted are zinc, magnesium, calcium, iron, and copper.

Stomach pain, frequent gas, bloating, and gastric reflux are all very common symptoms that could be caused by hypochlorhydria, or low stomach acid. Unfortunately, this condition is often mistaken for hyperchlorhydria, or excess stomach acid. Many people are given antacids or proton pump inhibitors that then exacerbate the problem. You can test for hypochlorhydria at home is two ways.

- Drink ½ cup water with 1 teaspoon of baking soda. If you have sufficient stomach acid, the baking soda will react with the acid in your stomach and form gas. If you burp within 10 minutes, you should have adequate stomach acid. If you do not burp at all, then this could be a sign that you have low stomach acid.

- Use pH strips and test your mouth pH first thing in the morning before breakfast. Eat breakfast and wait for half an hour before testing your mouth pH again. If the number has risen (for example from 6 to 8), then you most likely have adequate stomach acid. If the pH does not change, then you should take steps to increase your stomach acid. Test over multiple days to get a more accurate reading.

More formal tests can be done in conjunction with your healthcare practitioner. This includes taking a stool test to look for markers of undigested protein. Another method could be through a blood test.

HOW TO INCREASE YOUR ACID LEVELS

Here are some small steps you can take to holistically increase your stomach acid levels.

Chew thoroughly and eat small meals. Avoid drinking water during a meal, as it can decrease potency of stomach acid.

Eat more bitter greens. The bitter taste can stimulate stomach acid. Arugula, watercress, and mustard greens are all good choices.

Drink 1 teaspoon of apple cider vinegar with half a cup of water before each meal. You can gradually increase the amount of vinegar in a cup of water, up to 10 teaspoons. If you experience burning, immediately drink a glass a milk or take a teaspoon of baking soda in water.

Take digestive enzymes. Liz Lipski recommends plant-derived enzymes because they work both in the stomach and the intestines. Take one to two for a trial period of four weeks.

Take Swedish bitters. Bitters have often been used in Europe for digestion problems. They stimulate the production of HCL. Use in liquid form and take before meals.

Take betaine hydrochloride (HCL). Begin with one 10-milligram capsule before meals. Add one capsule at a time until you feel a warmth in your stomach. When you feel the warmth, take one capsule away and use for trial period of three weeks. If the warmth is uncomfortable, you can neutralize the acid with some baking soda and water.

Appendix C
GOODIES FROM GP INTERVIEWS

I'm so thankful that I had the opportunity to speak to many wonderful souls who helped me understand this disease on a more personal level and had great things to add. These are bits and pieces of interviews from the amazing soulful people that agreed to chat with me about their personal experience. There are two questions that I asked that I thought would be helpful to share: any tricks to help with flare-ups and advice for newly diagnosed folks. Hopefully, some of their tips resonate with you.

TRICKS TO HELP FLARE-UPS

"Pain-wise, a heating pad helps a lot. For nausea, peppermint can help for me. Using a bit of peppermint oil or sniffing an alcohol swab will sometimes take nausea away. A nurse once told me that I'm not the first person that said that. I have alcohol swabs everywhere. I will just open one and sometimes it will help with my nausea."

—Tabatha, 35, Indiana

"I take a bite of things throughout the day. A heating pad for pain helps. I exercise, which is difficult, but I feel like it helps keep things moving, and it helps my mental mood. I do take an herbal remedy called Iberogast, and if I take it while I'm eating, it seems to help with the pain."

—Melissa, 49, Indianapolis

"Something that I've discovered recently is a candied ginger chew, Gin Gins. I found this on a GP support group and lots of people were swearing by it. I have found a few of those helps to make it more bearable. Digestive tea helps with the nausea. Also, fresh mint helps sometimes. In water, it can be soothing."

—Jennifer, 29, New Brunswick

"Moving. I know it's painful, but any sort of gentle movement, just a short walk, it's helpful. Magnesium has really helped constipation. And lastly, going gluten free. I can't stress that enough."

—Tae-Lynn, 54, outside of Philadelphia

ADVICE TO NEWLY DIAGNOSED

"I want people to know that family and friends don't understand; they think of it as a temporary thing, and I want people to understand that this is serious and life changing. Be patient with yourself and find what is best for your own body."

—Melissa, 49, Indianapolis

"I would tell them to research the disease but not take in all the information that is out there online. It's a scary diagnosis. You can have mild to severe symptoms. Nobody can tell you how this disease is going to go. There is more reason to be hopeful than hopeless.

I would also tell them that you are stronger than this disease. You are not this diagnosis. You are still you. You are going to be able to handle this so that you can remember that you are still the person you were before this diagnosis.

In terms of medical care, I would say you need a motility specialist that specializes in gastroparesis. If your doctor tries to tell you they know how it will go, get a different one.

What has helped me is to be completely OK with whatever I can do that day. We ought to be like this before we are diagnosed. You have to give your best each day. If you are a mother and you have children you are still raising, and understand you gave the best you gave for that day, lay your head on the pillow and wake up the next day. Don't carry the guilt around; that stress that you are carrying around in your body is going to make the GP worse."

—Deb, 54, Arkansas

You can find out more about Deb's advocacy work at http://iamOKnow.com.

"You learn to find what works for you. Don't be scared to try; it doesn't mean you won't be able to eat again. Yes, I can eat, but I have to learn to make new things to love. I can find something that can taste just as good. You learn to adapt that way. It's a really big roller coaster, but it's important to not give up. I've wanted to throw in the towel. But I'm here, 11 years later, still working at it. I might not have the most adventurous life, but it's manageable.

Don't feel too scared, though it's easy to be overwhelmed. You need to find the right information out there. There are so many people who are newly diagnosed and they are terrified. They find out that they can die from this, but it's causing unnecessary panic. Someone who has 80 percent motility jumps to the worst-case scenario. A lot of people aren't there. Yes, things change at any time, but it can be a really manageable disease.

The last thing is that it's important to have a good GI doctor. One of the biggest barriers is the doctor. They don't believe you or are not willing to help. My GI fights tooth and nail for me. He literally saved my life. It's sad that sometimes the barrier for people is the doctor."

—*Jennifer, 29, New Brunswick*

"I would definitely say to consider alternative practices, not just what your medical doctor says. Look for a doctor that also knows they can't just send you home with a scrip in your hand and think that can solve anything. Look at the diet. Do a food journal. Everybody's body is different, the journal is key. I do have coffee in the morning, and if I do something else, it's apple cider vinegar in water. Talk to a nutritionist, or naturopathic doctor. There are other things out there that took me too long to discover."

—*Tae-Lynn, 54, outside of Philadelphia*

RESOURCES

BOOKS

Animal, Vegetable, Miracle: A Year of Food Life by Barbara Kingsolver

Clear Your Clutter with Feng Shui, by Karen Kingston

Fourfold Path to Healing: Working with the Laws of Nutrition, Therapeutics, Movement, and Meditation in the Art of Medicine by Thomas Cowan with Sally Fallon Morell and Jaiman McMillan

Full Moon Feast, by Jessica Prentice

The Garden of Fertility, by Katie Singer

Heal Your Body, by Louise Hay

The Life-Changing Magic of Tidying Up, by Marie Kondo

Lights Out: Sleep, Sugar, and Survival by T. S. Wiley with Bent Formby, PhD

The New Whole Foods Encyclopedia, by Rebecca Woods

Nourishing Traditions: The Cookbook that Challenges Politically Correct Nutrition and Diet Dictocrats by Sally Fallon Morell with Mary G. Enig

Omnivore's Dilemma: A Natural History of Four Meals by Michael Pollan

The Second Brain, by Michael Gershon

Why Zebras Don't Get Ulcers by Robert M. Sapolsky

Zapped: Why Your Cell Phone Shouldn't Be Your Alarm Clock and

1,268 Ways to Outsmart the Hazards of Electronic Pollution by Ann Louise Gittleman

ONLINE SUPPORT FORUMS

The Mighty
https://themighty.com

An online forum and magazine for those with disabilities, mental illness, and disease.

Inspire
https://www.inspire.com

Inspire is a forum with different communities where you can ask questions often and learn more.

FACEBOOK SUPPORT GROUPS

Gastroparesis Support Group: www.facebook.com/groups/GastroparesisSupportGroup

Gastroparesis Alliance: www.facebook.com/groups/gpalliance

WEB RESOURCES

Association of Gastrointestinal Motility Disorders
www.agmd-gimotility.org

A non-profit dedicated to all people with gastrointestinal motility disorders, including gastroparesis.

The Environmental Working Group (EWG)
www.ewg.org

An excellent resource is the Environmental Working Group, a consumer watchdog and political action organization that does its best to keep our food system clean and looks under the rug at products and foods that are available to the public. Their website includes the Dirty Dozen and Clean 15 guides, sunscreen and body care ratings, and grocery products ratings.

Oley Foundation
www.oley.org

The Oley Foundation was created to assist and enrich individuals reliant on intravenous nutrition and tube feeding. The site provides advocacy, educational, and networking resources.

The Story of Stuff
http://storyofstuff.org

This website and organization has great video resources on things that matter. What our consumerism does to the environment, what bottled water really is, toxicity of beauty products, plastics, and more. Wonderful for teachers and parents who want to engage children in learning how to better the economy and environment.

National Organization for Rare Disorder (NORD)
http://rarediseases.org/rare-diseases/gastroparesis

NORD has a well-written overview of gastroparesis, its treatments, and studies.

Aston Patterning Practitioners
http://www.astonkinetics.com/practitioners

Gastroparesis and Dysmotilities Association (GPDA)
http://www.digestivedistress.com/motility-rx

The archived GPDA site has in-depth descriptions of available treatments.

GASTROPARESIS-SPECIFIC WEBSITES

About Gastroparesis: International Foundation for Functional Gastroparesis Disorder
www.aboutgastroparesis.org

Gastroparesis: Fighting for Change
www.curegp.com

Emily's Stomach
emily-scherer.squarespace.com

Gastroparesis Crusader
Gastroparesiscrusader.weebly.com

Crystal Saltrelli, CHC
Livingwithgastroparesis.com

CONVERSIONS

VOLUME CONVERSIONS

U.S.	U.S. Equivalent	Metric
1 tablespoon (3 teaspoons)	½ fluid ounce	15 milliliters
¼ cup	2 fluid ounces	60 milliliters
⅓ cup	3 fluid ounces	90 milliliters
½ cup	4 fluid ounces	120 milliliters
⅔ cup	5 fluid ounces	150 milliliters
¾ cup	6 fluid ounces	180 milliliters
1 cup	8 fluid ounces	240 milliliters
2 cups	16 fluid ounces	480 milliliters

WEIGHT CONVERSIONS

U.S.	Metric
½ ounce	15 grams
1 ounce	30 grams
2 ounces	60 grams
¼ pound	115 grams
⅓ pound	150 grams
½ pound	225 grams
¾ pound	350 grams
1 pound	450 grams

INDEX

Vega protein powders, 73

Vegetables: fiber content, 155; organic, 80; skins, 66

Veggie broth, and food testing, 68; recipe, 92

Veggie Mineral Broth, 92

Vermicelli Noodle Soup, 108

Viral infections, as cause, 10

Visceral manipulation, 45

Vitamin B12, 21, 24, 71

Vitamins, 152-53; and birth control pills, 38

Vitamix blenders, 77-78

Volume conversions, 170

Wakame (seaweed), 83

Walking, 54-55

Water filters, 79

Water-soluble vitamins, 152

Weight conversions, 170

White miso, 79

Whole Chicken Broth, 91

Why Zebras Don't Get Ulcers, 47

Wood, Rebecca, quoted, 80-81

Yoga, 53-54

Yogurt Lassi, 142

Yucca, 96

Zapped, 52

ACKNOWLEDGMENTS

This book would not be possible without the insight and wisdom of those GPers that I interviewed. Thank you Allie, Melissa, Crystal, Tabatha, Trish, Deb, Jennifer, Tae-Lynn, and Sam. I hope that I was able to do your words and ideas justice, and I deeply appreciate your contribution.

I also want to thank all of my mentors and teachers from Bauman College and Three Stone Hearth, as well as all of my friends and family who have shown me little tricks and delicious recipes along the way. You have all influenced my life and education more than you know!

ABOUT THE AUTHOR

Born in Ohio and raised by Taiwanese parents, **Tammy Chang** now finds her home in the Bay Area. In addition to her health coaching work with clients and groups, she teaches fitness and is the head instructor at a capoeira school in Oakland.

Before being certified in holistic nutrition by Bauman College, Tammy received a BA in public policy from Duke University and as a New York City Teaching Fellow, received her MA in childhood education from Brooklyn College.

In her free time, she loves to roam the California forests and hot springs, sample restaurants, watch or read the latest sci-fi series, practice handstands, and spend time with family and friends.

Her first book, *The Nourished Belly Diet*, is available on Amazon; you can keep up with her via her website: www.thenourishedbelly.com